ACADEMIA OPHTHALMOLOGICA INTERNATIONALIS

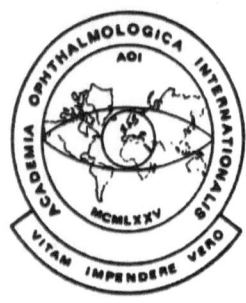

Board

President: GIUSEPPE SCUDERI
Vice-Presidents: BENJAMIN BOYD and RONALD LOWE
Secretary-General: PIERRE AMALRIC
Treasurer: JEAN-FRANÇOIS CUENDOT

History of Ophthalmology 5

Sub auspiciis
Academiae Ophthalmologicae Internationalis

Editor HAROLD E. HENKES
Geervliet, The Netherlands

Associate Editor CLAUDIA ZRENNER
Tübingen, Germany

Associate Editor DANIEL M. ALBERT
Madison, Wisconsin, USA

Springer-Science+Business Media, B.V.

ISBN 978-0-7923-2053-1   ISBN 978-94-011-2732-5 (eBook)
DOI 10.1007/978-94-011-2732-5

Documenta Ophthalmologica **81**: 1–16, 1992.

The history of stereoscopy

ROBERT A. CRONE

Department of Ophthalmology, Academic Medical Centre, Amsterdam, The Netherlands

Key words: History of ophthalmology, stereoscopy

Abstract. Ptolemy (127–148 AD) studied physiological diplopia, correspondence and the horopter. He had all the data to build a theory of depth perception through disparity detection, but left that undone. Alhazen (1000 AD) associated depth perception with the sensation of binocular convergence, just as Kepler (1611) and Descartes (1637). With the development of the concept of retinal correspondence and the fusion of the retinal images in the brain (Huygens 1667, Newton 1704) a cerebral mechanism of disparity detection became thinkable. The rise of Empiricism (Molyneux' Premise, the case of Cheselden) postponed the solution of the problem, finally reached by Wheatstone (1838). Physiological proof of Wheatstone's theory came from the experiments of Barlow et al. (1967).

The history of stereopsis is enigmatic. The amazing puzzle is this: why has its mechanism been discovered only 150 years ago while an adequate theory was within reach sixteen centuries earlier? In this article I will try to explain why the theory of binocular depth vision stagnated. The thinking on the perception of depth since the Scientific Revolution can easily be traced; it is more difficult for the period between the Greek civilization and the Renaissance.

The Greeks recognized that binocular single vision was a problem. By the simple trick of pressing a finger against one of the eyes, single vision could be interrupted. Therefore binocular vision was not self-evident and needed an explanation. *Galen* (129–179) thought that the images of both eyes were united in the chiasma, provided the eyes were in the straight position [1, 2]. He mentioned apparent size as a clue to distance. Galen, and none of the ancient scientists, associated perception of depth with binocular vision. That seems strange, the more so because Galen did notice that a near object during binocular vision was projected to two different places of the background. Evidently the Greeks never noticed that it was difficult to pass a thread through the eye of a needle with one eye closed. Although keen observers, the Greeks (as far as we know) never did the experiment to suppress depth perception by closing one eye. It should be noted that without such an experiment the superiority of binocular vision for depth perception is not all obvious: if you ask a number of naive observers whether the world looks different with one eye or with both eyes, the majority will answer the things look the same in both conditions. Binocular stereopsis is not the only clue to distance.

The Greeks could easily have done another experiment, as e.g. creating a sense of depth in a flat image. Although the making of a stereogram is extremely simple they did not make that discovery. Wheatstone, in 1838, made the first stereograms and was the first to prove that stereopsis was related to binocular vision. That corroborates the general truth that in science it is much more difficult to see a fairly obvious phenomenon as a problem, than to solve that problem.

Ptolemy

As far as we know the first and only Greek who thoroughly investigated binocular vision is the great astronomer *Claudius Ptolemy* (127–148), who wrote a book on optics [3, 4]. His problem is single vision, not depth perception. He analyzes physiological diplopia, the correspondence between both eyes, and even (without giving it names) the horopter and the cyclopic eye.

Ptolemy is an adherent of the 'extramission theory'. According to him vision comes about by the emission of visual rays from the eye. The rays issue conically from the centre of the eyes. The axes of the visual cones are the lines of fixation, where the visual acuity is highest. The lines of fixation correspond: when these visual rays meet at an object, the object is seen as one. Ptolemy places two rods in the median plane at different distances from the eyes. He discovers that during fixation of the distant rod the near rod is seen in crossed, heteronymous, diplopia. When the near rod is fixated the distant rod is seen in uncrossed, homonymous, diplopia. He notices that both rods are seen from an imaginary viewpoint which is located between both eyes. It is the 'cyclopic eye', a controversial concept which originated with the extramission theory [5].

The axes of the visual cones are not the only corresponding rays. Visual rays that make the same angle to the axes of the cones also correspond. They are *radii consimiles*. As a mathematician, Ptolemy must have known (although he does not mention it) that these corresponding visual rays intersect on a circle, drawn through the centre of the eyes and the fixation point, the so-called Vieth-Müller circle or geometrical horopter (Fig. 1).

In another chapter of his Optics Ptolemy returns to the problem of binocular single vision, when he discusses the theory of mirrors. He investigates which points in the periphery of the visual field are seen as single and comes to the conclusion that these points are situated in the frontal plane through the fixation point. (As his criterion was single vision, and not the modern criterion of equal visual directions in dissociated vision, his method was not sufficiently accurate to demonstrate that the 'horopter' was in reality a curved plane.)

Ptolemy gives his opinion about the perception of distance, but only for monocular vision. He thinks that distance can be estimated from the length

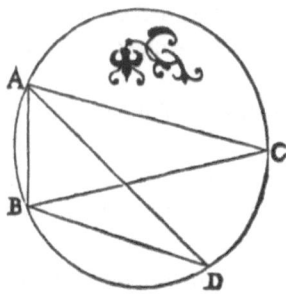

Fig. 1. Correspondence according to Ptolemy. The axes of the visual cones, with their apex in the eyes A and B meet at the fixation point C and are correspondent. Visual rays AD and BD, which make the same angle with AC and BC, also correspond. They meet on the geometrical horopter (the drawing is from Aguilonius, 1613).

of the visual ray between eye and object. He does not discuss binocular depth vision.

For Ptolemy the explanation of binocular stereoscopic vision was ready at hand. He knew that double images in front of the fixation point were crossed, and behind the fixation point uncrossed. He could have understood that crossed diplopia was synonymous with 'near' and uncrossed diplopia with 'far'. Had he realized that this criterion started to be valid even before diplopia became manifest (a nascent diplopia which we now call 'disparity'), then Ptolemy, and not Wheatstone, would have solved the mystery of stereopsis. Ptolemy knew nothing about image formation inside the eye, but the mechanism of stereopsis could have easily been formulated in terms of the psychological, phenomenal, space.

Ptolemy brushed past another important insight: Had he chosen the Vieth-Müller circle (and not the frontal plane) as the 'horopter', he would have concluded that all points seen as single and equidistant, would have been seen with a constant angle of convergence. Then he would have recognized the two pillars on which the doctrine of depth perception was going to be built in future centuries: disparity detection and convergence.

Alhazen and the perspectivists

Alhazen, the Arab scholar who lived about 1000 AD, was the first to construct an image of the visual world inside the eye. The image was upright and located in the lens. He shared Ptolemy's ideas about physiological diplopia, correspondence and binocular vision. To the psychological concept of corresponding visual rays he added a new, anatomical, concept: Corresponding elements inside the eye, points in the lenses with *positio consimilis*. Armed with this knowledge it is possible to trace lines from the object to the

4

Galenic centre of binocular vision in the chiasma. *Witelo* (Vitellio), one of Alhazen's epigones, made the drawing of Fig. 2, in his *Perspectiva* (1270, printed 1572 [6]).

For the perception of distance, Alhazen attached much importance to non-binocular clues such as apparent size, aerial perspective and parallax during head movements. However, he also mentions a binocular clue: the sensation of the degree of convergence of the eyes. It is an important new idea, later adopted by Kepler.

Alhazen was the father of the medieval students of the science of optics, the so-called 'perspectivists', such as Roger Bacon, Witelo and Peckham.

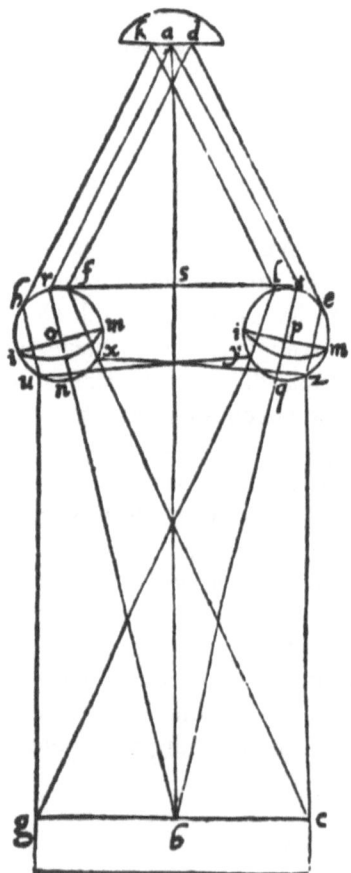

Fig. 2. A drawing from Witelo's Optics, Book III. The images of both eyes are fused in the chiasma.

Aguilonius

Aguilonius (1567–1617), a Belgian Jesuit scholar, has been regarded as the pioneer of binocular vision, but it seems more appropriate to call him one of the last of the perspectivists. His book on optics (*Opticorum Libri Sex*, 1613 [7, 8]), has been illustrated by his friend Peter Paul Rubens [9]. Aguilonius was well acquainted with binocular vision of depth. As a celibatarian priest he had to sew his own buttons and to pass a thread through the hole of a needle. As a child he had participated in a child's game that has been depicted by Rubens (Fig. 3). The instruction is, to touch a stick accurately with one eye closed. It is a task that is doomed to fail.

Aguilonius investigated physiological double images (fallacious images, *fallacii aspectus*) and the locus of binocular single vision in the same manner as Ptolemy. In the drawing by Rubens (Fig. 4) an old scholar looks at a frontoparallel plane. Cupids indicate the position of the fallacious images of a near object. Aguilonius coined the word *horopter*, literally: the limit of vision. In the horopter plane all vision rays end, leading to single vision or physiological diplopia. His horopter is not synonymous with our modern definition of the horopter as the locus of single vision or, even better, the locus of common visual directions. One could call it the 'projection of the cyclopic retina'. That, however, would have been an anachronism because Aguilonius did not yet know the function of the retina [10]. He never got hold of Kepler's rare book *Ad Vitellionem paralipomena* (1604 [11]), and still thought that visual perception came about in the lens.

Just as Ptolemy Aguilonius despised the circular geometric horopter (of which he makes a drawing in his book, see Fig. 1). He even explicitly

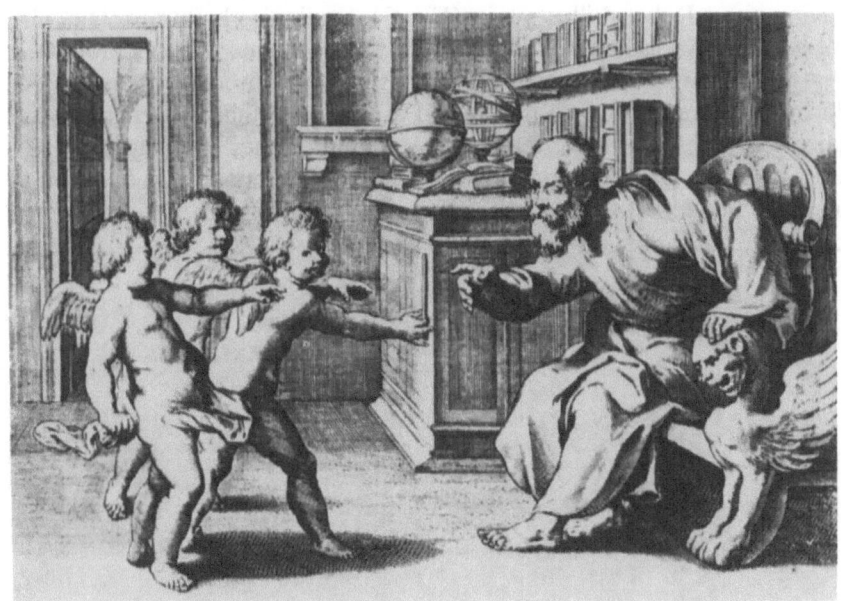

Fig. 3. The impossibility of depth discrimination with one eye (Aguilonius, Opticorum lib. III).

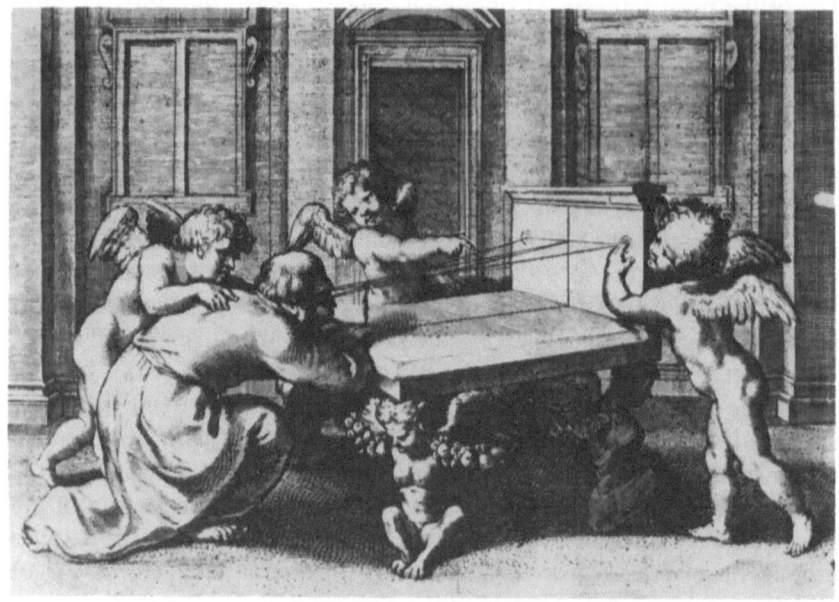

Fig. 4. Double images on the horopter plane (Aguilonius, Opticorum lib. IV).

rejected Alhazen's theory relating convergence to the perception of depth.

Having given Rubens' illustration (Fig. 3) Aguilonius had to explain why depth perception was better with two eyes than with one. Again he followed Ptolemy, believing that the length of the visual ray between eyes and object could be estimated. Then he introduced a new idea: that the length of the visual ray of one eye can better be judged by the other eye (Fig. 5).

Just as was the case with Ptolemy the theory of stereopsis slipped through Aguilonius' fingers. He failed to recognize the two possible criteria for the perception of distance: disparity and convergence.

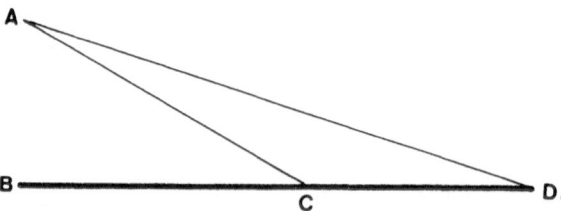

Fig. 5. The mechanism of binocular depth discrimination according to Aguilonius. The length of the visual ray from eye B to object C or D is estimated by eye A.

Kepler and Descartes

Johannes Kepler (1571–1630), the Imperial Mathematician of the German Emperor, proved in his celebrated book, *Ad Vitellionem Paralipomena*, that the eye made a flat and inverted image of the outer world on the retina. That discovery did not make the problem of stereopsis easier to solve, on the contrary! How was it possible to see depth in two flat images? We know the answer: the retinal images are not alike, and the small differences between the images can be detected. Kepler undoubtedly knew about the differences between the two images, but he must have considered it most unlikely that they could be detected. Vesalius had written that the optic nerves only approached each other in the chiasma, but did not have contact. Kepler accepted Vesalius' anatomical description, although he realized that the independence of the optic nerves was not conducive to binocular single vision (*Dioptrice*, 1611 [12]), let alone to the detection of minute differences of perspective.

As a matter of fact Kepler had another, very plausible, explanation of depth perception: *sensus communis distantiam notat ex sensu contortionis oculorum*, the 'common sense' perceives distance by feeling the rotation of the eyes (Dioptrice). It is Alhazen's theory of depth perception. *René Descartes* agreed with Kepler. His illustration in *La Dioptrique* (1637 [13]) shows a blind man who 'triangulates' distance with the aid of two sticks (Fig. 6). In the same way we triangulate distance with the convergence of our eyes. Kepler and Descartes did not discuss the sensory theory of depth vision by disparity detection; the motor theory of depth vision through convergence was satisfactory.

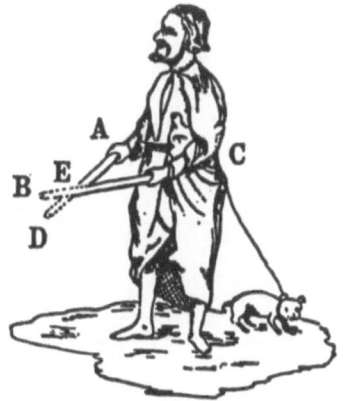

Fig. 6. According to Descartes we use our convergence to estimate distance, in the same way as a blind man uses two sticks.

Retinal correspondence

The problem of binocular single vision drew much attention in the seventeenth century. The first step was taken by the Dutch physicist *Christiaan Huygens*, who in 1667 defined corresponding retinal points [14]. A point in space, which is imaged on the centre of each retina, is seen as a single point. Retinal points in each eye with the same location in relation to the retinal centre, also correspond (Fig. 7).

Extremely interesting is the drawing (1672) of the French physicist *Jacques Rohault*, only three years after Huygens' formulation of corresponding points. Rohault postulated that, despite the non-crossing of the optic nerves, fibres from corresponding retinal points should meet somewhere at a higher level in the brain [15] (Fig. 8).

Isaac Newton had another hypothesis. He did not keep strictly to the teaching of Vesalius and presumed that fibres from corresponding points met in the chiasma and then proceeded to a final single locus in the brain. He published this hypothesis in the 15th query at the end of his book *Opticks* (1706 [16]): *Are not the species of objects united where the optic nerves meet before they come to the brain, . . . the fibres of the right side of both nerves uniting in the brain in such a manner that these fibres make but one entire picture?*

There is an original drawing of the hypothesis in one of Newton's manuscripts (Fig. 9). According to Newton the fibres of each eye 'united' to form one fibre [17].

That is a very satisfactory hypothesis to explain single binocular vision, but not detection of disparity. In this respect the diagram (Fig. 10) of the itinerant ophthalmologist *Chevalier Taylor* (1750), a younger contemporary of Newton, was better. According to him the fibres of each eye retained their individuality after semidecussation [18]. That was a prerequisite for the processing of disparity in the brain.

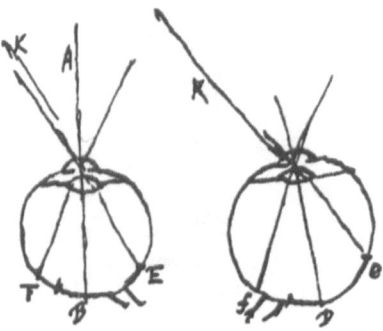

Fig. 7. Huygens' drawing of corresponding points. B and D are the principle corresponding points (later called the central foveae). F and f also correspond because the distances FB and fD are equal. The same is the case for BE and De.

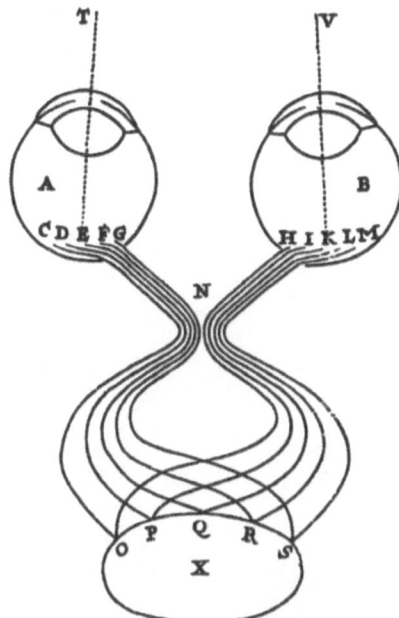

Fig. 8. The fusion of binocular images by a semidecussation of the optic fibres in the brain (Rohault).

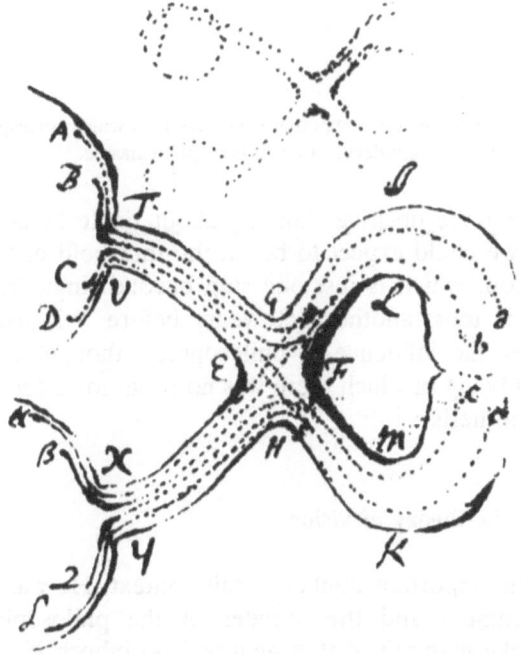

Fig. 9. Fusion of corresponding optic fibres in the optic chiasma (Newton).

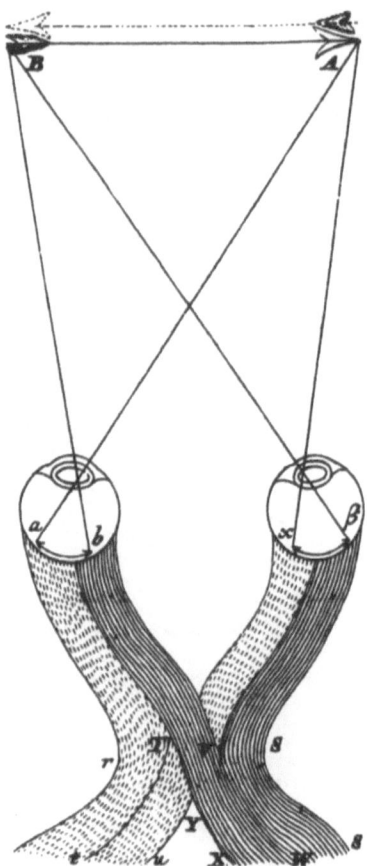

Fig. 10. A later drawing of Newton's hypothesis by Taylor, in which corresponding optic fibres keep their individuality after semidecussation in the optic chiasma.

At that moment the decisive thinking about single binocular vision had been done and we could expect to be on the threshold of the discovery of stereoscopic vision, which is just one step beyond single binocular vision.

Nevertheless it took another 150 years before Wheatstone made his discovery. Under the influence of philosophical thought a new theory of vision came into being in which there was no room for a further elaboration of Newton's hypothesis.

Empiricism and the theory of vision

John Locke is the important thinker in this context. He was the forerunner of the Enlightenment and the founder of the philosophical school of Empiricism. Locke maintained that man had no inborn ideas. Locke's aim was thus to reject the claims of the church and of the absolute monarchy, but his thesis also had a strong impact on the theory of knowledge. Locke rejected all *a priori* knowledge. He stated in his famous *Essay concerning Human Understanding* (1690) that all we know comes from experience. Man is originally like a piece of white paper, a *tabula rasa* [19].

The paragraph in Locke's Essay which is important for the theory of vision is the celebrated *Molyneux Premise*. Molyneux was an influential Irish politician and a student of the science of optics. He put the following question to Locke (I quote from Locke's Essay) about a man with congenital blindness who has been successfully operated for cataract at a later age. It was a 'thought experiment' because such hypothetical cases had not been described in reality. *Suppose a man born blind, and now adult, and taught by his touch to distinguish between a cube and a sphere. Suppose then the cube and the sphere placed on a table, and the blind man made to see. Quaere: whether by his sight, before he touched them, he could now distinguish and tell which is the globe, which the cube?*

Molyneux himself gives the following tentative answer: *Not. For though he has obtained the experience of how a globe, how a cube affects his touch, yet he has not yet obtained the experience that what affects his touch so and so must affect his sight so and so.*

Locke then continues: *I agree with this thinking gentleman, whom I am proud to call my friend.*

Only two decades after Locke's Essay *George Berkeley* [20] radicalized the teaching of Locke and published his *An Essay towards a New Theory of Vision* (1709). In its first paragraph he takes the reader in the midst of the problem: *1. My design is to shew the manner wherein we perceive by Sight the Distance, Magnitude and Situation of objects: also to consider the difference there is betwixt the ideas of sight and touch, and whether there be any idea common to both senses.* Then Berkeley comes immediately to the point: *2. It is, I think, agreed by all that Distance, of itself and immediately, cannot be seen.*

Berkeley defends the thesis that the sensations of the various senses have nothing to do with each other. Smells and sounds have nothing in common. The same is true for the sensations of vision and touch. The eyes produce sensations of light and colour, touch teaches us spatial relations. The eyes are not able to see depth or other spatial relations unless an empirical relation is established between vision and touch.

Berkeley's philosophical position was spiritualistic. He denied the existence of matter and held the opinion that the world consisted of nothing but sensations and sensing spirits (God's spirit included). Berkeley's influence was immense because his thinking satisfied everybody. He satisfied the free-thinkers by his radical empiricism and the conservatives by his pious spiritualism. Finally he even became a bishop.

His authority became unassailable after a case report by the London

ophthalmologist *William Cheselden* (1728 [21]): *An Account of some Obser-*
vations made by a young gentleman, who was born blind, or lost his Sight so
early, that he had no Remembrans of ever having seen, and was couche'd
between 13 and 14 Years of Age.

The result of the cataract operation was at first disappointing: *When he*
first saw, he was so far from making any Judgement about Distances, that he
thought all Objects whatever touch'd his Eyes ... He knew not the Shape of
anything, nor any one Thing from another, however different in Shape, or in
Magnitude; but on being told what Things were, whose Form he before knew
from feeling, he would carefully observe, that he might know them again.

It took some time before he learned to distinguish shapes. To see depth
he needed the initial help of touch. But all's well that ends well: *A Year after*
first seeing, being carried upon Epsom Downs, and observing a large
Prospect, he was exceedingly delighted with it, and call'd it a new Kind of
Seeing.

Berkeley, and all empiricists after him, considered this case report as the
decisive proof of the theory of Locke and Molyneux. There is certainly no
medical case in history that made a greater impression. *Voltaire* described it
in 1738 in his *Elémens de la philosophie de Newton*, a book that made no
lesser stir in the world than Darwin's Origin of Species. *Diderot*, the
principal author of the Encyclopédie, amply discussed the case in his much
read *Lettre sur les aveugles*, in 1749. Another encyclopédiste was the
naturalist Buffon. For *Buffon* [22] vision was the handmaid of touch. Touch
was, in Buffon's eyes, the geometrical sense. Vision had much to learn from
touch. It had even to unlearn bad habits. I cite his own words, in English
translation [23]. *Before touch teaches the true position of objects and their*
own bodies, children see top and bottom reversed: their eyes mislead them as
to the true positions of objects. A second defect of vision at this stage is to
represent objects doubly, for each eye forms its own image of the same object.
Only experience with touch can rectify this error, which it does so well that we
eventually believe we see objects single and upright, and we credit this
impression to sight, when it actually comes from touch.

Such was the ideological atmosphere in the psychology of vision. No
specialist in the theory of vision would have thought of considering depth
vision as a specific visual mechanism. The idea of disparity induced stereopsis had to come from a brilliant outsider, not from a philosopher or a
psychologist.

Charles Wheatstone

The physicist Charles Wheatstone did more than just inventing the stereoscope (Fig. 11). He immediately realized the theoretical background of his
findings. Even in his first article (1838 [24]) on the stereoscope he wrote: *No*
doubt some law or rule of vision may be discovered which shall include all the

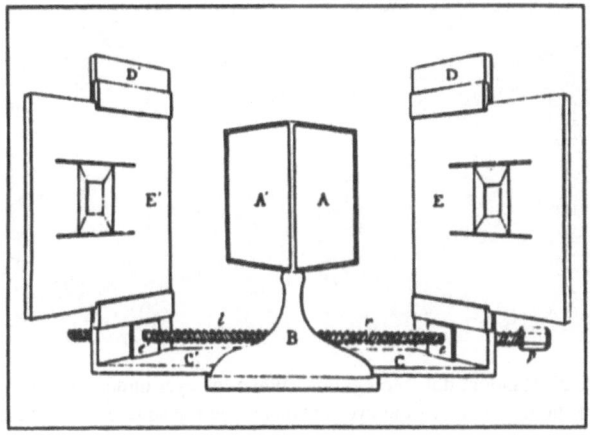

Fig. 11. Wheatstone's stereoscope.

circumstances under which single vision by means of non-corresponding points occurs.

His discovery initiated the fall of empiricism and the rise of nativism in visual science. Empiricism, however, offered a strong resistance, even until the second half of this century. Wheatstone, for that matter, himself still supposed that the art of seeing depth from disparity was taught by experience. *Helmholtz*, in many respects a follower of Locke, held the same opinion. In his Handbuch (1867 [25]) he tells an odd tale of a childhood memory: *I remember passing under a church tower. On the gallery beneath the top of the tower I saw people, which I mistook for dolls. I begged my mother to give me one of those, thinking she could easily reach for them.*

It is impossible to take this account seriously outside the intellectual landscape of empiricism.

In the fifties of this century American psychologists still had much trouble to get rid of the fallacy that touch teaches vision. It needed – among other experiments – the test with the 'visual cliff' [26] (Fig. 12) to convince

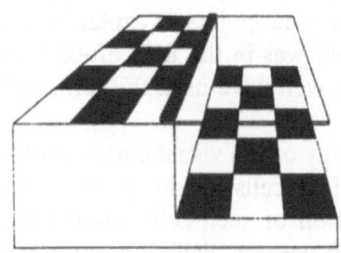

Fig. 12. The visual cliff. A baby refuses to crawl from the left to the right side of the glass plate.

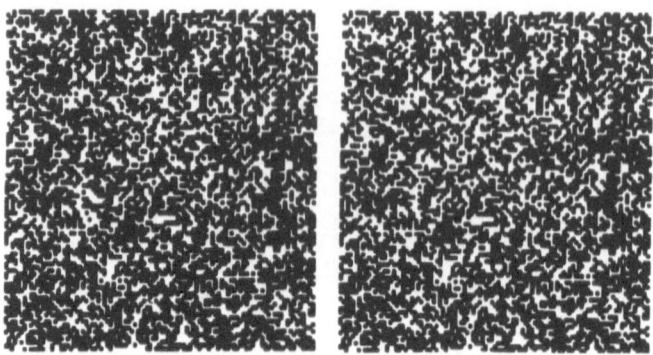

Fig. 13. Bela Julesz' 'Random dot stereograms'. When the eyes underconverge a central square is seen in front of the paper; when the eyes overconverge the square is behind the plane of the paper.

psychologists that it was not necessary for a child to fall off a roof to learn that the street is lower than the roof.

That depth discrimination is an original visual ability has been demonstrated convincingly and elegantly by *Bela Julesz* (1964 [27]). His 'random dot stereograms' (Fig. 13) elicit a sensation of depth without prior identification of an image and thus without prior experience. Disparity detection must be a very elementary visual process which occurs at an early stage of visual processing.

The neurophysiology of stereoscopic vision

That that is indeed the case, was demonstrated by *Barlow, Blakemore and Pettigrew* (1967 [28]), who disclosed the neural mechanism of depth discrimination. With the technique developed by Hubel and Wiesel they registered the action potentials of binocular cortical cells. Many binocular cells only responded when the stimuli were presented at a certain disparity (Fig. 14, from Bishop [29]). For the first time since Ptolemy stereopsis entered the domain of physiology. (It is true that Wheatstone used the theory of corresponding retinal points to explain the binocular perception of distance. But his discovery was in the field of experimental psychology, and Wheatstone could just as well have used the term *radii consimiles* instead of 'corresponding points'.)

Had the neurophysiology of the visual cortex evolved in a totally different manner, binocular cortical cells might perhaps have been called by a different name. Stimulation of such cells might have elicited convergence, and the same cells which we now call disparity detectors might have been called 'convergence generators'. That would have pleased Descartes, the first physiologist who tried to understand the actions of the body without

15

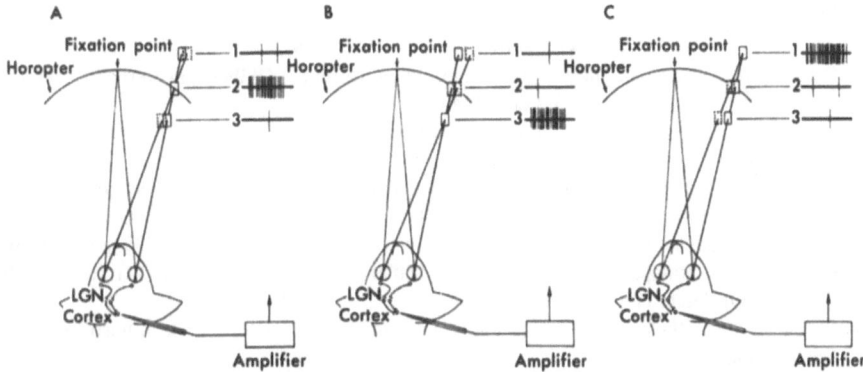

Fig. 14. Bishop's simplified drawing of cortical disparity detection. In the cases B and C a binocular cell responds only when the visual stimulus is in front of, respectively behind the horopter (LGN: lateral geniculate nucleus).

involving the soul. Descartes [30] was interested in the reflex arc (Fig. 15), the bridge built on an afferent and an efferent pier. There are good reasons to assume that depth vision can be reduced physiologically to a reflex arc in which in-coming and out-going signals exactly correspond: perceived disparity can be measured in fractions of a minute of arc, but the same is true for convergence. It is not unthinkable that the efferent theory of depth perception (of Alhazen, Kepler and Descartes) will eventually also be founded on a solid physiological basis.

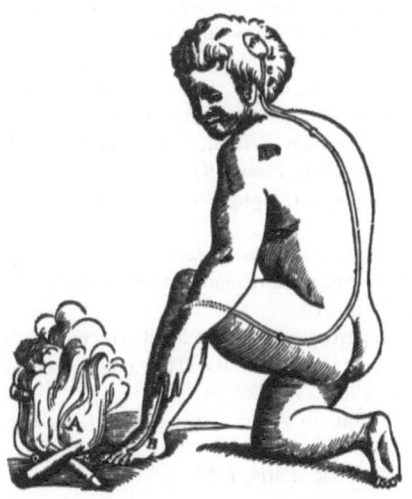

Fig. 15. Descartes' reflex arc.

16

References

1. Doesschate G ten. De derde commentaar van Lorenzo Ghiberti in verband met de middeleeuwse optiek. Thesis Utrecht 1940.
2. Lindberg DC. Theories of Vision from Al-Kindi to Kepler. Chicago: The University of Chicago Press, 1976.
3. Lejeune A. Euclide et Ptolemée. Deux stades de l'optique géométrique grecque. Louvain: Université de Louvain, Recueil de travaux d'histoire et de philologie, ser. 3, fasc. 31, 1948.
4. Lejeune A. Les recherches de Ptolemée sur la vision binoculaire. Janus 1958; 47: 79–86.
5. Crone RA. A noncyclopean diagram of binocular vision in strabismology. Graefe's Arch Clin Exp Ophthalmol 1988; 226: 113–116.
6. Witelo. Opticae thesaurus. Ed. F. Risner, Basel 1572. Reprint New York: Johnson Reprint Corporation, 1972.
7. Aguilonius F. Opticorum libri sex. Antwerpen, 1613.
8. Rohr M von. Auswahl aus der Behandlung des Horopters bei Fr. Aguilonius um 1613. Z ophthalmol Optik 1923; 11: 41–59.
9. Jaeger W. Die Illustrationen von Peter Paul Rubens zum Lehrbuch der Optik des Franciscus Aguilonius, 1613. Heidelberg: Verlag Brausdruck GmbH, 1976.
10. Ziggelaar A. François Aguilón, S.J. (1567–1617), Scientist and Architect. Roma: Institutum Historicum S.I., 1983.
11. Kepler J. Ad Vitellionem paralipomena, quibus astronomiae pars optica traditur. 1604. In: Johannes Kepler: Gesammelte Werke, Ed. Walther von Dyck and Max Caspar, München, 1939.
12. Kepler J. Dioptrice. 1611. In: Ges. Werke, loc. cit.
13. Descartes R. Discours de la méthode . . . plus la Dioptrique, les Météores et la Géometrie. Leyde, 1637.
14. Huygens C. Deuxième complément de la Dioptrique (1667). In: Œuvres Complètes, XIII/2. La Haye, Nijhoff, 1916.
15. Rohault J. Traité de physique. Amsterdam, 1672.
16. Newton I. Opticks. London, 1704.
17. Grüsser O-J. Vom Ort der Seele. In: Aus Forschung und Medizin 1990; 5(1): 75–96.
18. Taylor J. Mechanismus des menschlichen Auges. Frankfurt, 1750.
19. Locke J. An Essay concerning Human Understanding. London, 1690.
20. Berkeley G. An Essay towards a New Theory of Vision. London 1710.
21. Cheselden W. An account of some observations made by a young gentleman, who was born blind, or lost his sight so early, that he had no remembrance of ever having seen, and was couched between 13 and 14 years of age. Roy Soc Philos Tr 1728; 35: 447–450.
22. Buffon N. Histoire naturelle de l'homme. Paris, 1749.
23. Morgan MJ. Molyneux' Question. Vision, Touch and the Philosophy of Perception. Cambridge: Cambridge University Press, 1977.
24. Wheatstone C. Contributions to the physiology of vision. Roy Soc Philos Tr 1838; 128: 371–394.
25. Helmholtz H von. Handbuch der physiologischen Optik. Leipzig, 1867.
26. Walk AD, Gibson EJ. A comparative and analtyical study of visual depth perception. Psychol Monogr 1961; 75, nr 519.
27. Julesz B. Binocular depth perception without familiarity cues. Science 1964; 145: 356–362.
28. Barlow HB, Blackemore C, Pettigrew JD. The neural mechanism of binocular depth discrimination. J. Physiol 1967; 193: 327–342.
29. Bishop PO. Binocular Vision. In Adler's Physiology of the Eye. St. Louis, C.V. Mosby Comp., 1987.
30. Descartes R. Traité de l'homme. Paris, 1664.

Address for correspondence: Prof. Dr R.A. Crone, Reguliersgracht 1, 1017 LJ Amsterdam, The Netherlands.

Documenta Ophthalmologica **81**: 17–25, 1992.

Helmholtz, the first reformer of ophthalmology*

HAROLD E. HENKES

Eye Clinic, Rotterdam, The Netherlands

Key words: History of ophthalmology, Helmholtz

Helmholtz' invention of the ophthalmoscope in 1850 was a case of serendipity, the gift of being able to make discoveries by pure accident. The theory of the glow seen in the pupil of the eye in the dark was formulated by Helmholtz' friend and colleague Brücke, who observed this phenomenon while studying the eyes of their mutual friend, Emil du Bois-Reymond (1818–1896; Fig. 1). Brücke, du Bois-Reymond and Helmholtz were very close friends; all three were physiologists and about the same age, at the time of Helmholtz' invention and they lived in or near Berlin.

Brücke saw du Bois-Reymond's pupil lit up by a red glow, but did not think to ask himself about the path of the emergent rays of light from du Bois-Reymond's retina. Helmholtz (1821–1894; Fig. 2) however, who wanted to explain to his students at the Army Medical School the phenomenon of the red reflex from the fundus of the eye, constructed the path the optic rays take from the retina of the test person to the observer's eye. He then suddenly became aware of the immense implications of an instrument by means of which the reflected light could enter the observer's eye unhampered, forming an image on the retina and thus allowing the study of the fundus of the living human eye. In a few days Helmholtz had constructed a provisional instrument which he called an ophthalmoscope (Fig. 3).

In contrast with the foregoing, the construction of the ophthalmometer (Fig. 4), as Helmholtz called his invention a few years later, in 1855, was not a case of serendipity. Helmholtz, who, like Donders, his Dutch counterpart, started his career as a poor army surgeon, was from his early years greatly interested in physics and mathematics. His aim was to construct an instrument which would allow the exact measurement of the optical constants of the living eye, that is to say: the curvatures of the cornea and the lens surfaces, thereby elucidating the states of refraction and accommodation. He designed a perfect instrument, but its use was difficult and time-consuming. A special room of sufficient dimensions was even needed.

* Helmholtz Memorial Lecture held at the opening ceremony of the IXth Congress of the Societas Ophthalmologica Europaea, Brussels, May 1992.

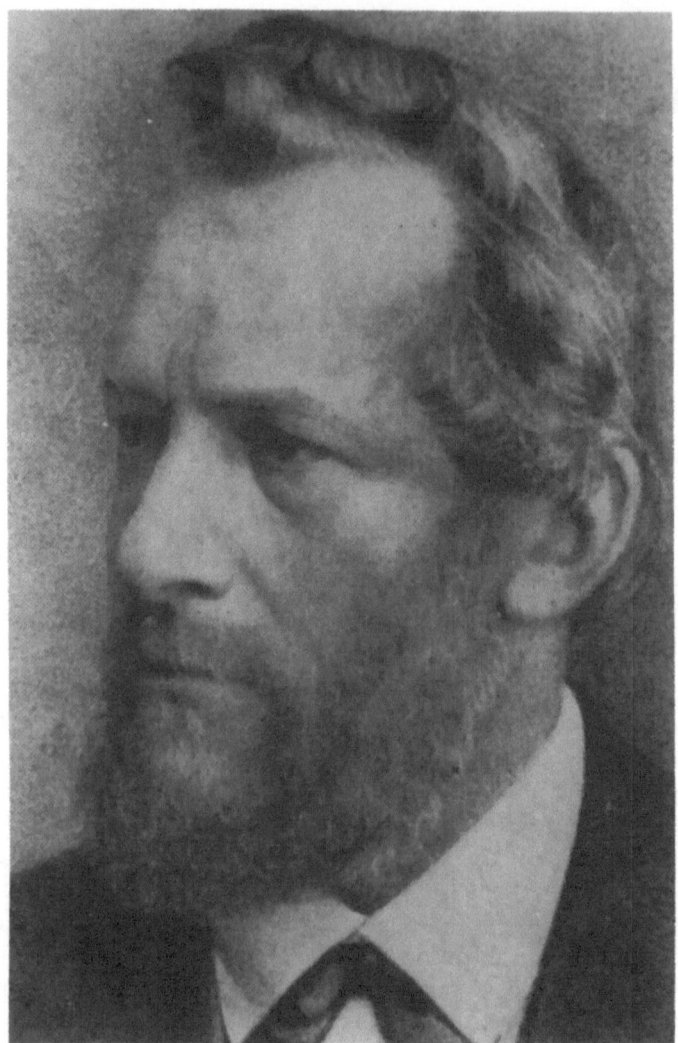

Fig. 1. Emil du Bois-Reymond (1818–1896).

It is to the credit of Coccius, the professor of ophthalmology at Leipzig, that he grasped the implications of this purely scientific instrument for the ophthalmologist's practice. In 1867 Coccius modified Helmholtz' ophthalmometer into an instrument which had the potential for use in practice for the measurement of the curvature of the cornea. But only after Javal in 1881, with the aid of Schiøtz, had adapted Coccius' construction (unfortunately without mentioning Coccius' name), was an instrument created which allowed the measurement of the corneal curvature in a simple way. From then on, the astigmometer of Javal/Schiøtz made its way worldwide into the

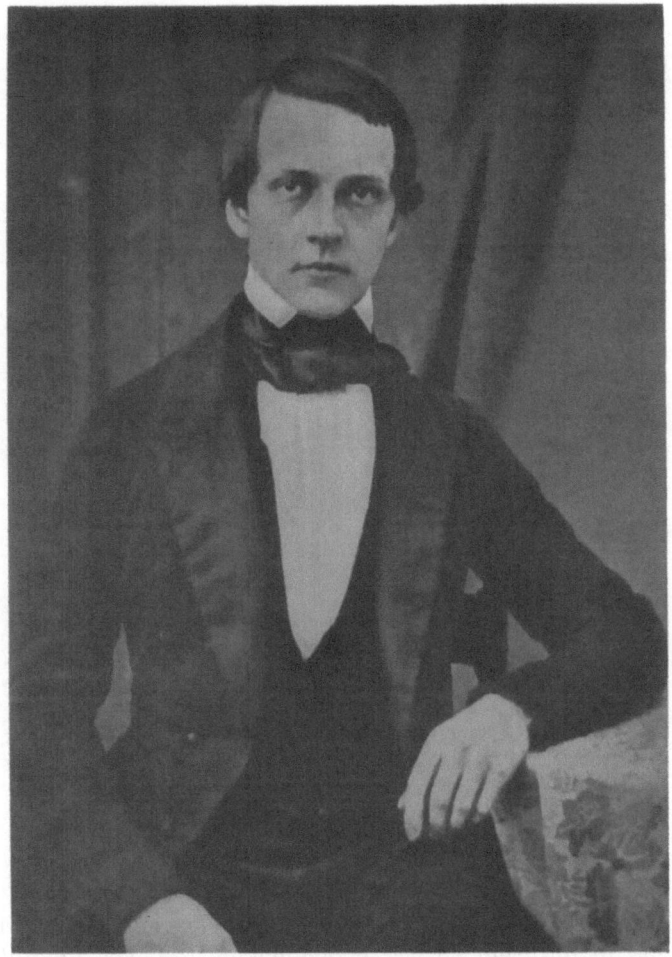

Fig. 2. Hermann Helmholtz (1821–1894) at the age of 26.

ophthalmologist's consulting room. Figure 5 shows an astigmometer constructed in the nineties by the Dutch instrumentmaker Kagenaar, but
electrified around 1900.

Helmholtz' third major contribution to ophthalmology is certainly his *Handbook on Physiological Optics*, which was written between 1856 and 1866.
The three parts: Die Dioptrik des Auges (Dioptrics of the Eye); Die Lehre
von den Gesichtsempfindungen (Visual Sensations), and Die Lehre von den
Gesichtswahrnehmungen (Visual Perceptions) truly merit Von Graefe's
dictum: 'the Bible of the ophthalmologist'.

But Helmholtz interest in scientific problems went far beyond the field of
physiological optics alone. While his handbook was an inexhaustible
source of information for ophthalmologists, physiologists and even physic-

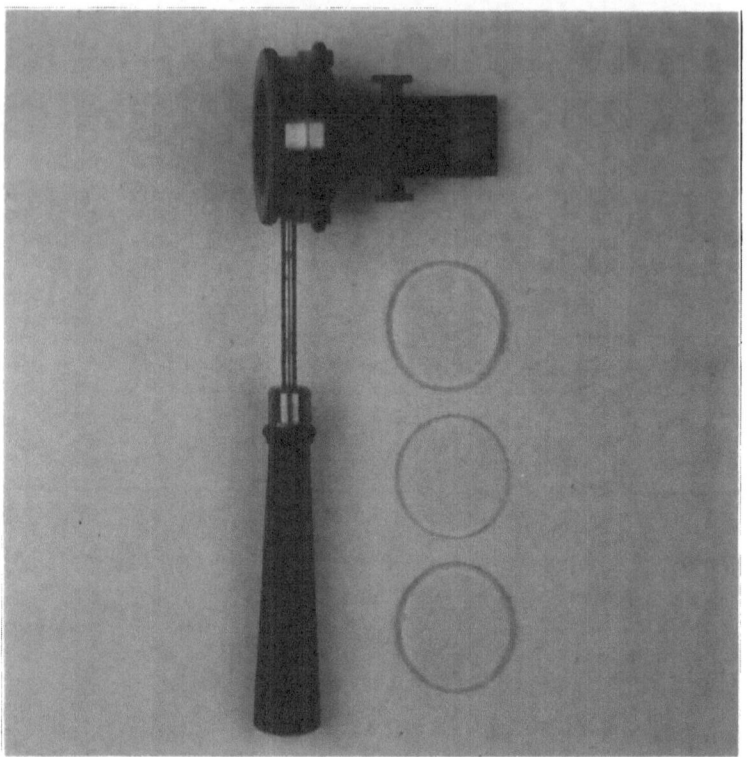

Fig. 3. The first model of the ophthalmoscope.

ists, after the publication of part 1, he turned his attention in 1856 to acoustics, and in this field he was epoch-making too. His *Physiologische Grundlagen zur Theorie der Musik* (Physiological Principles of the Theory of Music), and later his *Lehre von den Tonempfindungen* (The Principles of Tone Perception, 1862) became the daily handbooks and compulsory reading of not only audiologists, physiologists and physicists, but musicians and music-loving amateurs as well. Mr. Steinway for instance, in the 19th century already famous for the quality of his grand pianos, visited the Helmholtz family regularly. He discussed the suggestions Hermann Helmholtz gave him and tried out the improvements on the grand piano in the home of the Helmholtz family.

Meanwhile Helmholtz, in 1852, had published his studies on the speed of nerve conduction. Helmholtz was the first person who was able to measure latency times in milliseconds thanks to the construction of a special kymographion (Fig. 6). He discussed his results with his longtime friend, Emil du Bois-Reymond, who was at that time already a famous Prussian physiologist, and who devoted a great deal of his life to the study of 'animal electricity', on which subject he published in 1849 his famous book entitled:

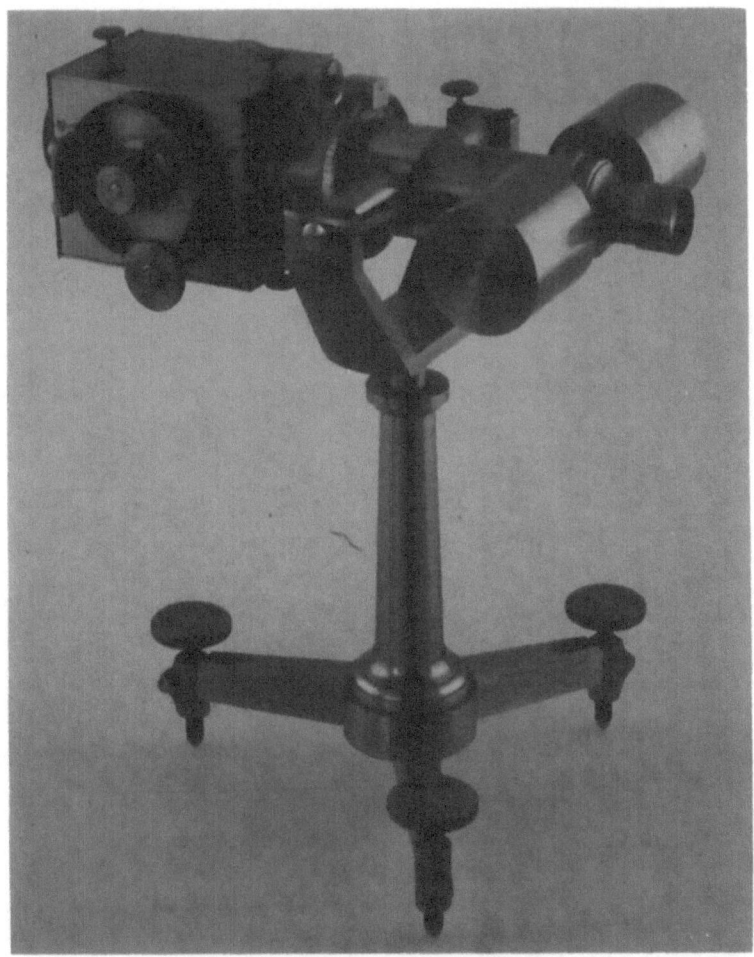

Fig. 4. Helmholtz's ophthalmometer.

Untersuchungen über thierische Elektrizität. By the way, Du Bois-Reymond is the discoverer of the standing potential of the eye, on which the present-day routine recording of the EOG is based.

It goes without saying that Helmholtz was a distinguished guest at many scientific meetings. He was acquainted with a host of interesting people. He was a friend of Bowman, but also of Faraday, Tyndall, Wheatstone; he dined with Gladstone, attended a dinner party with Charles Dickens as table president and complained in March 1864 that the smog in London is so bad, that even in full sunshine, the sun is dark red.

But Helmholtz was much too busy to attend medical congresses, although he was a doctor himself. He liked to visit fellow-scientists in their own laboratories. Attending large meetings was a waste of time in his opinion;

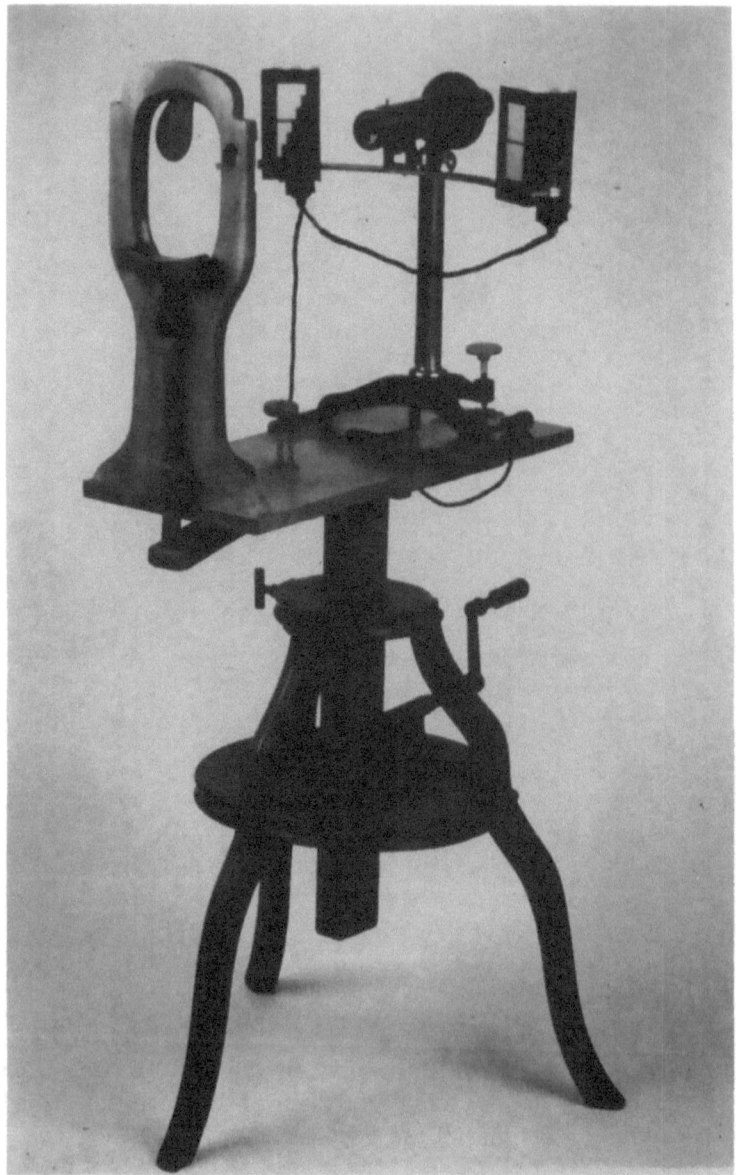

Fig. 5. An astigmometer of Javal/Schiøtz built by Kagenaar, instrumentmaker of Donders in Utrecht, Netherlands. This model of the nineties was electrified around 1900.

real progress came from personal encounters. But in Paris in 1867, during a world exhibition, he attended the international ophthalmology congress. At that time he visited Knapp, Liebreich and other internationally famous ophthalmologists. And at the official dinner in Paris he was toasted with:

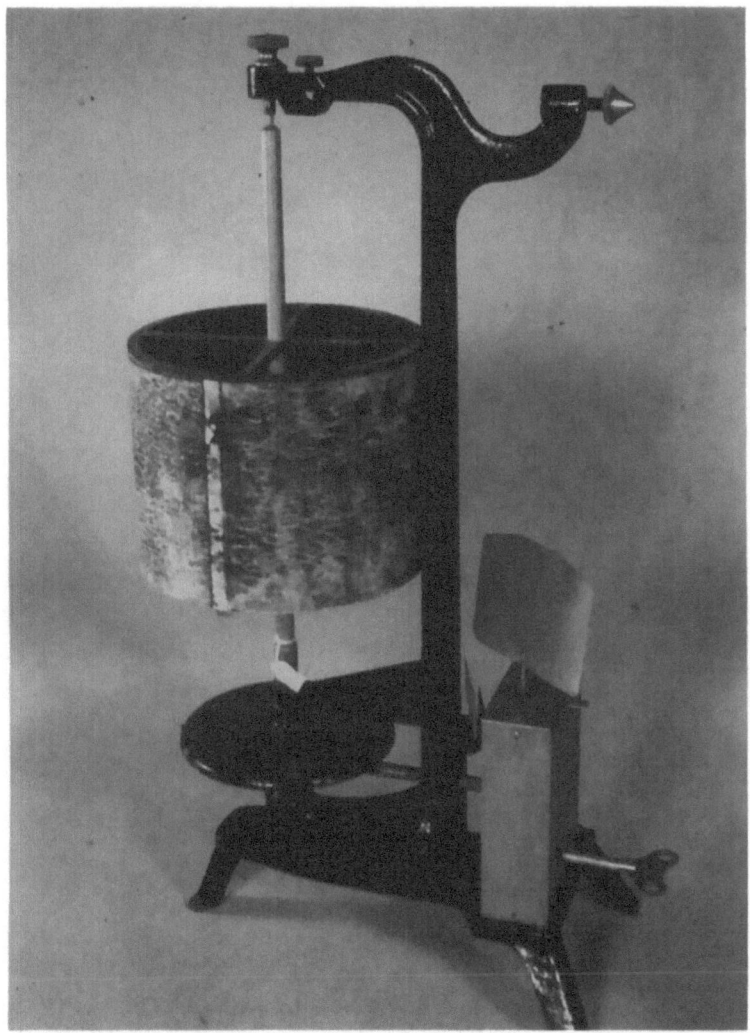

Fig. 6. Kymographion of the second half of the nineteenth century.

'L'ophtalmolgie était dans les ténèbres – Dieu parla que Helmholtz naquit – Et la lumière est faite!'. He visited the German club of ophthalmologists in Paris too and lectured at their meeting. Helmholtz was a friend of Mendelssohn-Bartholdy with whom he travelled through France and Spain.

Finally, one other aspect of Helmholtz' versatility should be mentioned: his deep interest in nature. But always with a certain aim: to understand the way in which nature behaves. He studies and explains to lay audiences natural phenomena such as the origin of glaciers, as he did to this fellow-travellers after boarding a Swiss post chaise through the mountains. He

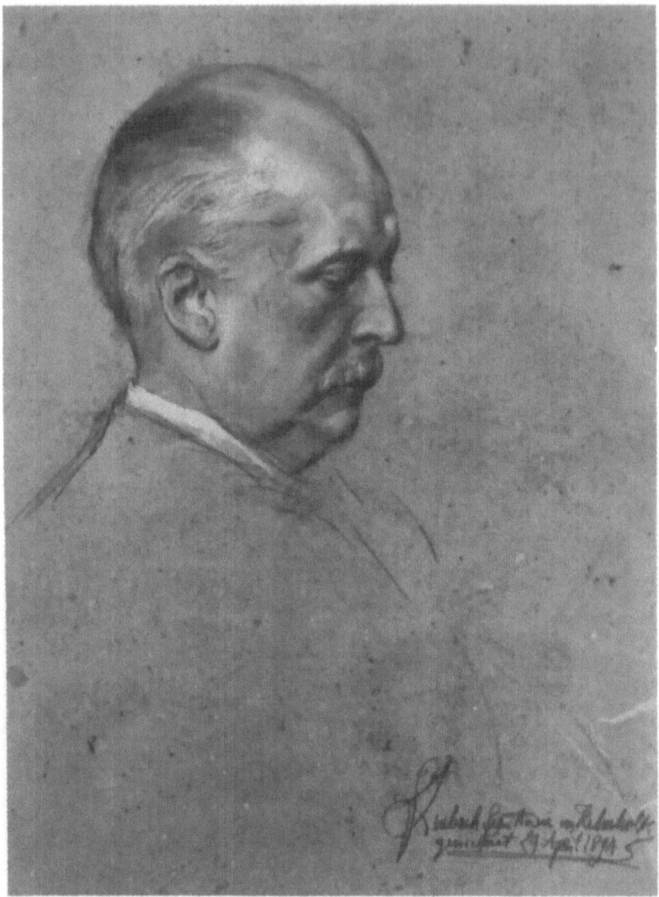

Fig. 7. Hermann von Helmholtz in 1894.

occupies himself with problems of wave and cloud formations, storms, hurricanes and volcanic eruptions; he descends into Mount Vesuvius, sails the seas between Scotland and Ireland in a small boat, studying wave formations, seasick but determined. Helmholtz occupies himself with weather forecasts, discusses aerodynamics in relation to the problem of how to steer balloons, etc. Indeed, Hermann von Helmholtz (Fig. 7), as he was called after he was knighted in 1883, was a versatile thinker and most probably the foremost scientist of the second half of the 19th century.

Von Helmholtz was the pivot around which the scientific world of the second half of the 19th century turned; the central figure to whom scientists came and went. In due modesty I suggest that the Dutch artist Escher has recorded something of this sort in his special way (Fig. 8). Creatures, be it frogs or ophthalmologists, returning from the scientific feeding-grounds at the centre of the world, making way for others who have not yet been so fortunate.

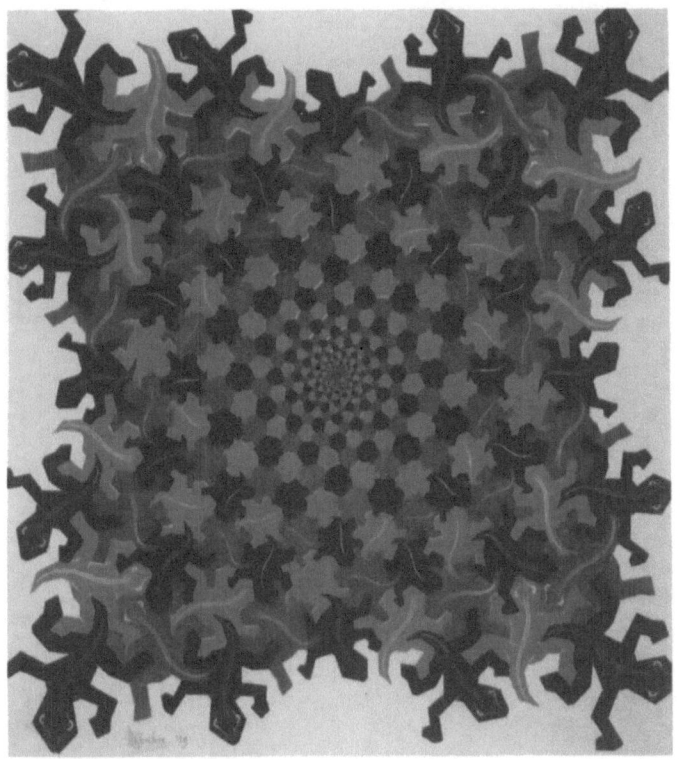

Fig. 8. 'Development II', 1939, M.C. Escher (1898–1972).

Note

Most data mentioned by the author are to be found in the biography of L. Koningsberger: *Hermann von Helmhotz*, published in three volumes in 1902/1903 and in *Anna von Helmholtz, ein Lebensbild in Briefen*, published by her daughter, Ellen von Siemens-Helmholtz, in two volumes in 1929.

Address for correspondence: Prof. Dr Harold E. Henkes, Landswerf 1, NL-3211 BR Geervliet, Netherlands.

Documenta Ophthalmologica **81**: 27–35, 1992.
© 1992 *Kluwer Academic Publishers*.

Christoph Scheiner's eye studies

FRANZ DAXECKER

University Eye Clinic, Innsbruck, Austria

Key words: History of ophthalmology, physiological optics, Scheiner's experiment

Abstract. Christoph Scheiner was born in 1573 or 1575. In 1595 he entered into the Order of the Jesuits; he died in 1650. In 1619 his book *Oculus*, dealing with the optics of the eye, appeared in Innsbruck. The invention of the telescope was of utmost importance for progress in astronomical and physical research. Scheiner himself built telescopes and discovered the sunspots. As a result, an unpleasant priority dispute with Galilei ensued. From 1624 onwards, Scheiner was in Rome, where his main work *Rosa Ursina* was published in 1630. A part of this book deals with the physiological optics of the eye as well. Some of his discoveries and experiments are taken from these two books: determination of the radius of curvature of the cornea, discovery of the nasal exit of the optic nerve, increase in the radius of curvature of the lens in case of accommodation, Scheiner's procedure (double images with ametropia), refractive indices of various parts of the eye, Scheiner's experiment. Without any doubt, Christoph Scheiner belongs to the foremost scientists of the first half of the 17th century.

Introduction

The Jesuit mathematician, physician and astronomer, Christoph Scheiner (ca. 1573–1650) stood, together with others, at the beginning of modern scientific thinking. Nikolaus Copernikus picked up the ideas of Aristarchus of Samos (fl. ca. 270 BC), first to maintain that the Earth rotates and revolves around the sun, and developed his new teachings: not the earth is the centre of planetary movements, but the sun. Tycho Brahe could not yet decide to accept the heliocentric theory and created his own system. According to Tycho Brahe, the planets moved in orbits around the sun, while the sun and the planets as a whole moved round the stationary earth at the centre of the universe [1]. Due to the achievements of Galilei, the Copernican, heliocentric system was developed further.

At that time, the invention of the telescope was of great importance for the progress in astronomical and physical research. Religious unrest shook the people of the 16th century, the Thirty Years' War, starting in 1618, devastated large parts of Europe.

This was the time of the Swabian Jesuit Father Christoph Scheiner (Fig. 1). The life and work of this man were not always appreciated sufficiently in public, the fame of posterity was rather inclined towards his contemporaries Kepler and Galilei. In many ways, the anti-clerical and anti-Jesuit rational-

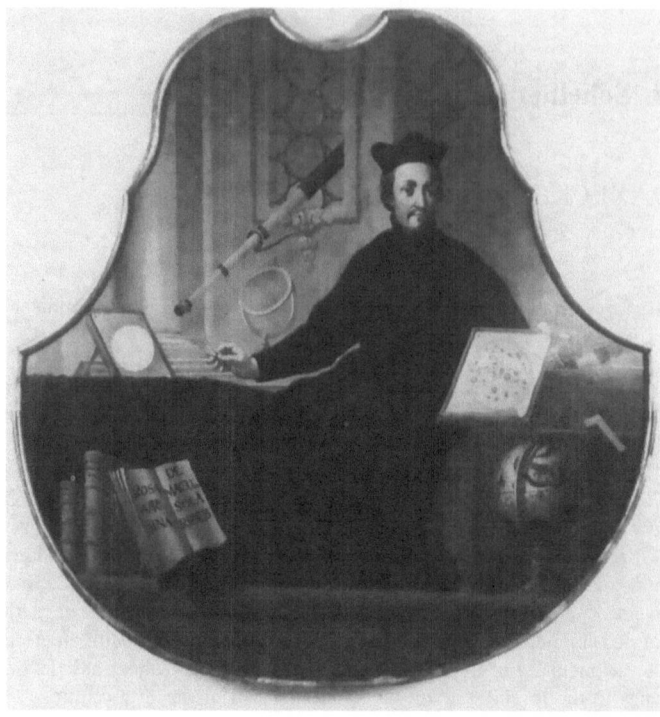

Fig. 1. Christoph Scheiner SJ. Through the telescope, the sun rays project the picture of the sun onto a screen. In the left hand, Scheiner holds a drawing with sunspots (Stadtarchiv-Municipal Archives, Ingolstadt).

ism passed over Scheiner's scientific achievements. Scheiner defended the principle of the primacy of observation: 'Against a single, true, observed fact a thousand hair-splitting arguments are without any value at all' [7]. Scheiner counts amongst the most important scientists in the first half of the 17th century. He was able to combine practical skill in the building of instruments with the power of observation. Because of his research, he won the favour of many Catholic sovereigns and was thus able to contribute towards the spreading of his order. In his interpretation of the cosmos, he stuck to forcing the geocentric system and not the Copernican or Galileian hypothesis. Very likely, his ecclesiastical office and the not yet completely provable hypothesis did not permit him to represent the new system [2]. In 1603 he invented the pantograph (stork's bill), built an astronomical telescope, equipped with two lenses, for which he cut the lenses himself [3], and drew the first map of the moon for the German speaking part of the world [4]. In 1611 Scheiner discovered the sunspots, he determined the rotation time of the sun and the position of its equator. As a result, an unpleasant priority dispute between himself and Galilei arose. As from 1624 onwards, Scheiner was in Rome. He was (in an unjustified manner) accused of having been involved in the trial against Galilei [5]. In 1615 he dedicated the paper *Sol ellipticus*, dealing with the elliptical shape of the sun when rising and when setting, to the Archduke Maximilian of Tyrol. This Archduke, Maximilian, the German Master of the Teutonic Order, received a telescope in 1615 which had the defect of representing all objects the wrong way round. Father Scheiner improved the instrument and henceforth the Archduke was able to watch all wordly objects in an upright position. In 1619, his book

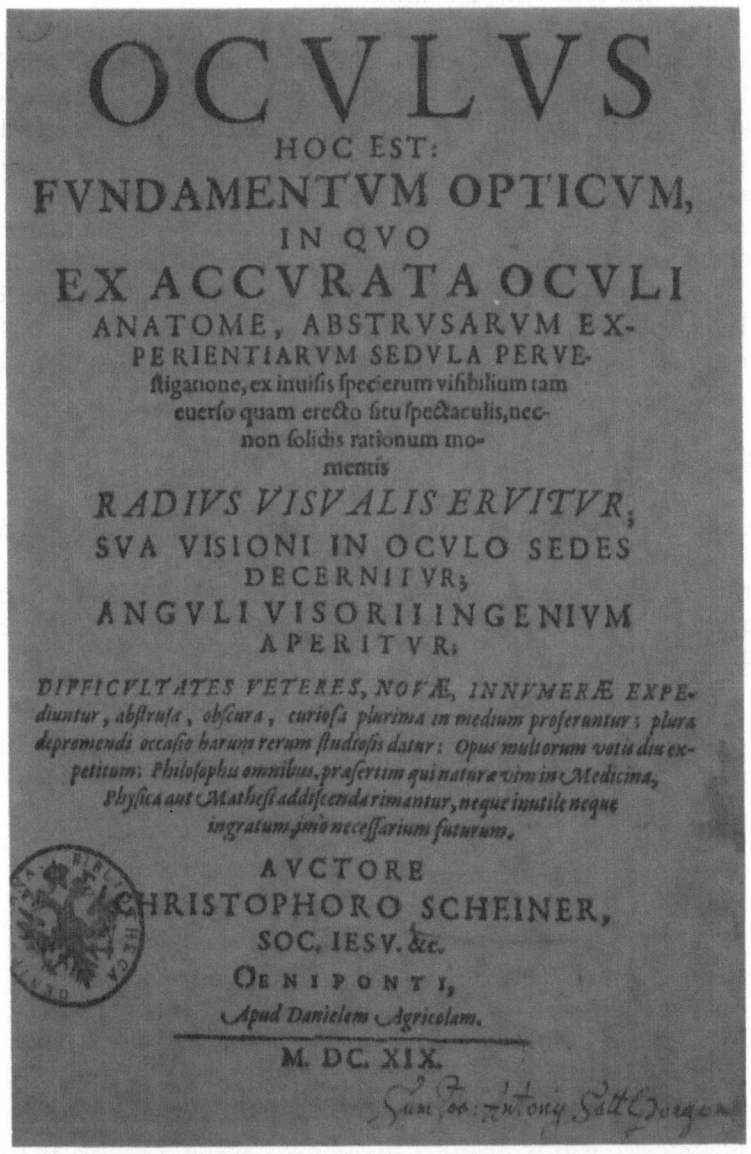

Fig. 2. Scheiner's book "Oculus", printed in Innsbruck by Daniel Bauer in 1619.

Oculus hoc est: Fundamentum opticum [6], dealing with the physiological optics of the eye (Fig. 2), was published in Innsbruck. His main work, *Rosa Ursina sive sol* [7] – an important work on the sunspots, was written in Rome in 1630. In the second volume of this work, he compares the optics of the eye as 'natural tube'. These two books form the basis of the following considerations.

Curriculum vitae of Christoph Scheiner

Christoph Scheiner was born on July 25th of the year 1573 or 1575 in Wald near Mindelheim in the Bavarian part of Swabia. There do exist different data on the year of his birth [8, 9, 10]. In 1595 he entered into the Order of the Jesuits in Landsberg. After completion of his theological and philosophical studies, he became professor for mathematics in Ingolstadt from 1610 onwards; from 1616 to 1620 he served as adviser to Archduke Maximilian and subsequently to the latter's successor, Archduke Leopold, in Tyrol. After short stays in Freiburg/Br., Vienna, and Neiße, he lived in Rome from 1624 until 1633; subsequently he stayed in Vienna, and in 1636 he returned to Neiße, where in 1650 a stroke put an end to his life full of work.

Christoph Scheiner's contributions to physiological optics

Scheiner's discoveries and experiments relative to physiological optics found in his treatises *Oculus* and *Rosa Ursina* are discussed in the following. The author draws upon both the original Latin text (see Notes) and the German translation (11). The figures (xylographs) originate from *Oculus* and are reproduced in the original size.

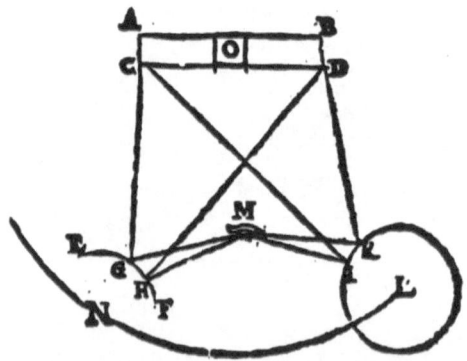

Fig. 3. The window A, B, C, D is projected onto the cornea, in particular onto G, H and equal to these are I, K on the glass ball L at the same distance of the eye from M.

1. Radius of curvature of the cornea

Scheiner realized that the sclera does have a flatter radius of curvature than the cornea and he was also able to prove this by an experiment. He held two glass balls next to the eye, the window projected therefrom was then to be seen in the same size both on the cornea and on the glass ball. With this experiment, Scheiner demonstrates the first step towards the development of an ophthalmometer. He writes in this connection in *Oculus* (page 13): Keep a number of glass balls of exactly the same globular shape ready, regardless whether they are hollow or full. With their help you are able to determine the size of the cornea (curvature) of any eye (Fig. 3).[1]

2. Nasal exit of the optic nerve

Until Scheiner it was assumed that the optic nerve enters into the eye at the rear pole opposite the pupil; this error was corrected by him (page 17) [13, 14, 15]. Figure 4 shows this representation.

3. Hint of an increase in the radius of curvature of the lens in case of accommodation

On page 23 he states that the ciliary processes are endowed with a certain movement capacity: . . . . , through which the entire eye either extends or shortens and the fluids themselves move at least the crystal lens and the vitreous body forward and backward, as well as flatten the shape of the crystal lens a little or make it more spherical.[2] This is a hint to the fact that Scheiner has not only observed a displacement of the lens, but also an alteration in the shape of the lens for the purpose of accommodation.

4. Light reaction of the pupil

Here, Scheiner indicated an experiment for the proof of the reaction of the pupil (page 30): Put any person at a place illuminated by a bright light like

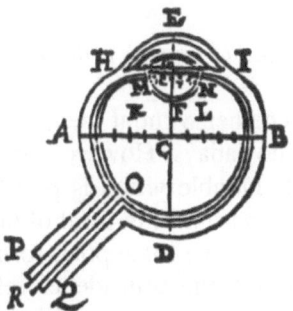

Fig. 4. Exact representation of the parts of the eye, the optic nerve enters excentrically into the eye.

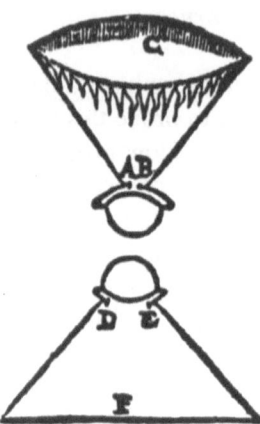

Fig. 5. A, B denominates the narrow pupil, E the wide pupil, C the bright light, F the darker place.

the sun, direct his eye towards you and the light, have a look at it and you will notice that immediately after that the pupil is no bigger than a small lens, frequently even smaller. Lead this person away from that bright place to a darker one, watch his pupil at the same time and you will see that it extends virtually with each individual step (Fig. 5).[3] According to M. von Rohr [11], the light reaction was possibly already known to Leonardo da Vinci.

5. Narrowing of the pupil in case of accommodation

Scheiner describes an experiment (page 31) with which he proves the narrowing of the pupil in case of accommodation. He writes in this connection: Take a small needle or something similar into your hand, keep it away from the eye looking onto the pin-head and move it gradually towards the eye so that it is hardly a finger's width away from it; simultaneously with the approach of the needle to the eye, the latter's pupil will close, simultaneously with the distance, it will open (Fig. 6).[4]

6. Scheiner's procedure – double images with ametropia

One cannot speak about Scheiner without mentioning the experiment which is still known by his name nowadays. However, he was not yet in a position to explain this experiment. Double vision is possible only, if the beam of rays originating from the object unites in front of or behind the retina, since two separate images of one and the same point form through the two holes. This principle was applied with the coincidence refractometer, in a similar way also with many photographic cameras and telemeters; double images are used for adjustment criteria [12]. With respect to this point he writes

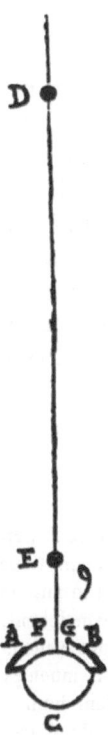

Fig. 6. The pupil A, B narrows to the size F, G when the needle approaches from D to E.

(page 37): Take a small circle A, B, C, cut from a thin layer (a metal sheet is as a rule more suitable for this purpose), where the eyelet A, D. C protrudes. Provide this small circle with two openings by means of a needle, as you please, at E and F, when the distance E and F is to be smaller than your pupil. Following that, close one eye and bring the other one as closely as possible to the holes and do look simultaneously through both holes at spires during the daytime and at either brighter stars, the moon and the sun, or candles and torches set up in the distance (in distances of 10 or 20 steps or more) during the night-time. You will then see everything double and more clearly than when you watch it without hindrances.[5] Scheiner was myopic [11, 16], he had noticed the stenopeic effect here.

7. Refractive indices of the various parts of the eye

He determined the refractive indices of eye fluids (page 64) and of the lens by filling bottles and small bottles, blown ball-shaped, with aequeous humour or vitreous body, sinking them into water and observing whether under these circumstances small objects, pushed underneath these bottles, do cause a magnification.

8. Scheiner's experiment

This experiment is mentioned by him in his book *Rosa Ursina*; in *Oculus* (1619 edition) no reference is made to it [13]. He writes in this connection: that the radiations do cross each other by the way before the picture of the object appears on the retina Y Z, I have not only proved by many very obvious experiments and reasons in my work *Oculus*, but I have also seen it very clearly here in Rome in the jubilee year (1625), when after removal of the sinew skin at the bottom of the eye, the light falling in from a candle stroke the retina with crossed rays. This experiment was made by me several times with many animal eyes (*Rosa Ursina*, page 110).[6]

Notes

1. In promptu habeto multos globulos vitreos perfectè sphaericos seu cauos, siue solidos, perinde est, horum beneficio magnetudinem tunicae Corneae oculi cuislibet sic explorabis.
2. Praesertim Crystallinum & Vitreum vel in anteriora vel posteriora compellant: figuramque Crystallini nonnihil vel attenuent, vel conglobent.
3. Statue hominem quemuis in locum luce vehemente, vtputa solari illustrem, oculumque contra te & lucem statutum considera, & inuenies pupillam subinde lenticula non maiorem, imo frequenter minorem; hunc eundem hominem sensim è loco illo lucido subduc in obscuriorem, simulque in pupillam intende, & eandem ad singulos quasi passus dehiscentem aspicies.
4. Altera Experientia est haec: Accipe in manum aciculam, aut quid simile eamq; ab oculo in aciculae caput intento remotam tene, sensimq; ad oculum admoue; ita vt crassitie digit vix absit; vna cum accessu aciculae ad oculum tuum claudetur pupilla eiusdem, van cum recessu ab eodem aperietur.
5. Accipe orbiculum ex lamina aliqua tenui excisum (metallica huic vsui fere aptior est) A B C, es quo ansula A D C promineat. Hunc transfige acu duobus foraminibus vbi libet ad E & F, intertuallo E F, minore, qua sit tua pupilla: quo facto, altero oculorum clauso, alterum ad foramina facta applica vicinissimè, & per ambo simul turrium fastigia de die, aut stellas luculentiores, de nocte, lunam, solémue vel auersas procul candelas, lampadas, ad passus (10, 20, aut amplius) contemplare; videbis omnia geminata, & quidem distinctiùs, quam si ea absque vllo obstaculo considerares.
6. Caeterum decussationem radiorum, fieri antequam imago obiecti in Retina, Y Z effigietur, non tantum in Oculo meo mutis euidentissimis experimentis atq; rationibus demonstraui, sed etiam in oculo humano hic Romae anno iubilaeo apertissime vidi, vbi abrasa in fundo oculi sclerode, immissum candelae per pupillam lumen radijs decussatis in tunicam Retinam accidit: id quod in multis brutorum oculis saepius expertus eram.

References

1. Mason SF (1972). A History of Sciences, New rev. ed. New York: Colliers book.
2. Rösch H. (1959). Christoph Scheiner: Lebensbilder aus dem Bayerischen Schwaben. München: Hueber, pp. 183–311.
3. Goercke E. (1990). Christoph Scheiners Ausführungen über Glaslinsen und ein moderner Nachahmungsversuch. Die Sterne 66 (6): 371–379.

4. Goercke E. (1988) Christoph Scheiners Mondkarte und die frühe Selenographie. Die Sterne 64 (4): 229–236.
5. Ziggelaar A. (1986). Scheiner und Grassi Widersacher Galileis. Physica didactia 13: 35–43.
6. Scheiner Ch. (1619). Oculus hoc est: Fundamentum opticum. Oeniponti, Apud Danielem Agricolam.
7. Scheiner Ch. (1626–1630). Rosa Ursina sive sol. Braccioni, Apud Andream Phaeum Typographum Ducalem.
8. Braunmühl A. (1891). Christoph Scheiner als Mathematiker, Physiker und Astronom. Bamberg: Bayerische Bibliothek, Band 24.
9. Duhr B. (1913) Geschichte der Jesuiten in den Ländern deutscher Zunge. Freiburg: Herdersche Verlagshandlung.
10. Koch L. (1934). Jesuitenlexikon: Die Gesellschaft Jesu einst und jetzt. Paderborn: Bonifazius.
11. von Rohr M. (1919). Ausgewählte Stücke aus Christoph Scheiners Augenbuch. Zeitschrift für ophthalmologische Optik 7: 35–44, 53–64, 76–91, 101–113, 121–133.
12. Schober H. (1972) Verfahren zur Bestimmung der Sehschärfe und der Korrektur von Fehlsichtigkeit. In: K. Velhagen (ed.), Der Augenarzt, Band 2. Leipzig: Georg Thieme Verlag.
13. Hirschberg J. (1908). Geschichte der Augenheilkunde. In: Graefe Saemisch Handbuch der gesamten Augenheilkunde, Band 13. Leipzig: W. Engelmann.
14. Kölbing MA. (1967). Renaissance der Augenheilkunde 1540–1630. Bern Stuttgart: Verlag Hans Huber.
15. Mauthner L. (1876). Vorlesungen über die optischen Fehler des Auges. Wien: W. Braumüller.
16. von Rohr M. (1920). Zur Würdigung von Scheiners Augenstudien. Archiv f. Augenheilk. 86: 247–263.

Address for correspondence: Ass.-Prof. Dr. Franz Daxecker, University Eye Clinic, Anichstr. 35, A-6020 Innsbruck, Austria.
Tel. (512) 504 3731; Fax: (512) 504 3722.

Documenta Ophthalmologica **81**: 37–42, 1992.

Jules Janssen (1824–1907): From ophthalmology to astronomy

PIERRE AMALRIC
Centre Médical Ophtalmologique, Albi, France

Key words: History of ophthalmology, Jules Janssen, ophthalmoscopy

Jules Janssen was born into a cultivated family but he was the first to enter into the medical or physical science. His father was a musician of Belgian descent and his maternal grandfather was the architect Paul-Guillaume Le Moyne. An accident in his early childhood left him permanently lame. Consequently he was educated at home and never attended school. He studied music with his father but financial difficulties obliged him to go to work at the age of sixteen. While working for a bank from 1840 to 1848 he was able to complete his education and earn a baccalaureate degree at the age of twenty-five. Janssen attended the University of Paris, receiving his *licence ès science* in 1852. He then obtained a post as substitute teacher in a lycée.

During that period, in the middle of the 19th century, ophthalmology was emerging as a medical specialty in no small part due to new discoveries in optics. Janssen became the friend of the French scientists Giraud-Teulon, Follin and Nachet who were particularly interested in optical problems.

Janssen's first scientific work was a study of the absorption of radiant heat in the optical media of the eye (*Sur l'absorption de la chaleur rayonnante obscure dans les milieux de l'oeil. In Annales de Physique et de Chimie, 3rd series, 60: 71–93*). He showed that the optic media are transparent only for visual rays and that the focalization of the thermal radiation has no harmful effect on the retina because nine tenths of the radiation is absorbed. This carefully executed work was also based on experimentation involving eyes of animals. Here he studied absorption of the rays by the cornea, the lens and the other ocular structures. This work earned him a doctorate of science in 1860. In his thesis, he wrote:

> . . . having often had the opportunity to be present during the tapping of blast furnaces, I noticed that the radiation from the bath of molten metal . . . in no way affects the eyes; thus, one can follow without fatigue the various phases of the operation if one takes the precaution of protecting the face with a mask that exposes only the eyes. As absorption by the optic media appeared to me to be an important physiological fact, I proposed to verify and measure it by precise experiments.

But, as concerns our speciality, Janssen's main contribution is related to ophthalmoscopy. With Follin of the Faculty of Medicine, he introduced

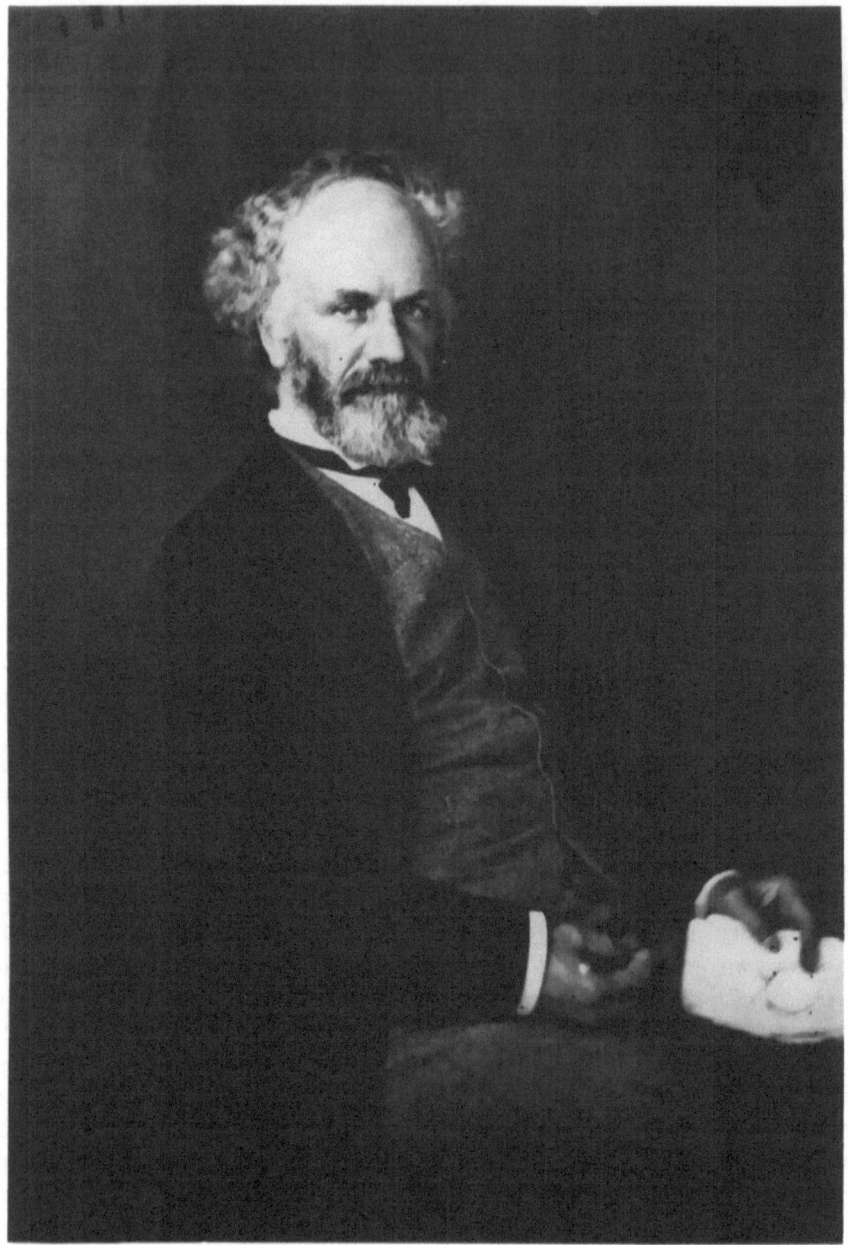

Fig. 1. Jules Janssen (1824–1907).

some modifications in the design of the ophthalmoscope in order to ensure safe and efficient observation of the fundus. Janssen worked out a system of observation with coloured filters which only kept the green light which was considered the least dangerous for the eye.

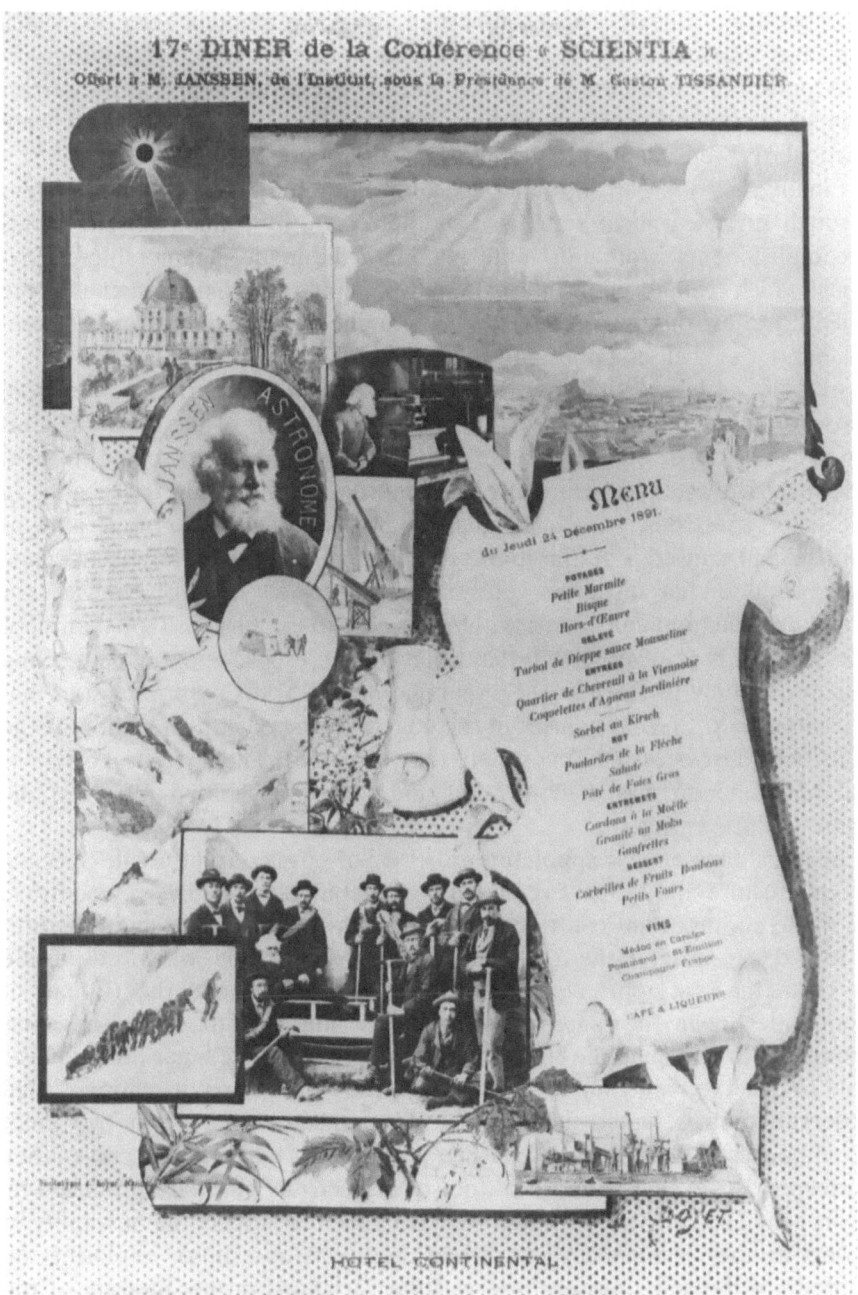

Fig. 2. This menu symbolizes all of Janssen's life. From left to right: (1) Creation of the observatory of Meudon, (2) In 1870, during the Franco-Prussian war, departure from Paris in a balloon to observe an eclipse in Algeria, (3) Spectrographic studies of the luminous rays, (4) Creation of the observatory at the summit of Mont Blanc, and (5) Janssen among his porters from Chamonix.

A picture of this device was published at the Academy of Sciences, which indicates that Janssen's modifications dealt with the system of lighting.

Around the same period, Janssen carried out experiments on the refraction of the cornea and on keratoconus. He designed lenses which were particularly well adapted to compensate for irregular astigmatism.

Finally, he took part in numerous studies on the quality of luminous rays through diverse optical systems. But that was only a minimal part of his accomplishments, from 1861 until his death, he made innumerable discoveries which gained him international recognition. His researches were oriented to astronomy, architecture, art, archeology, and eventually mountaineering, as well as optics and ophthalmology.

In 1861, as he was in Paris with Follin working on the ophthalmoscope, Janssen mounted a small observatory on the flat roof of the house that his wife owned north of Montmartre. Here he began to work on a problem posed by Brewster in 1833 concerning the nature of certain dark bands in the solar spectrum, bands irregular in presence and most noticeable at sunrise and sunset. For this purpose, Janssen constructed a spectroscope possessing a high dispersive power and furnished it with a device for regulating the luminous intensity. He was able to establish in 1862 that these spectral bands resolve into rays and that their presence is permanent. On a mission to Italy in the following year, he demonstrated with precision that the intensity of the rays varies in the course of the day as a function of the density of the terrestrial atmosphere they traversed. The terrestrial origin of the phenomenon was demonstrated and Janssen proposed for them the name 'telluric rays'.

In 1865, Janssen was appointed professor of physics at the Ecole Spéciale d'Architecture and, after several astronomical missions in diverse countries, he made an important contribution to the knowledge of the solar structure.

In order to observe the total eclipse of 18 August 1868, which was visible in India, he was sent by the Academy of Sciences and the Bureau of Longitudes near the Bay of Bengal. His aim was to study the solar prominences. Keeping the slit of the spectroscope on the lunar limb, he was able to observe highly luminous spectra while the sun was in eclipse. Visual observation in a finder showed that these spectra came from two great prominences. Janssen measured the position of the brightest rays: they corresponded to rays C and F of the solar spectrum which are produced by hydrogen. The brightness of the rays led Janssen to suspect the possibility of observing the prominences even when there was no eclipse. Exploring the contour of the sun, Janssen observed the variations in the intensity of the line and the modifications in its structure, he also demonstrated that other bright lines appear, all of them corresponding exactly to the dark lines of the absorption spectrum:

> Thus was demonstrated the possibility of observing the lines of the prominences outside of eclipses, and of finding therein a method for studying these bodies (Annuaire du Bureau des Longitudes 1869: 596).

From 18 August to 4 September Janssen carried on his observations on the unobscured sun for 17 days after the eclipse, and established maps of the prominences. He continued his observation in the Himalayas and on 25 December he wrote that the solar photosphere is surrounded

> ... by an incandescent atmosphere, the general, if not exclusive base of which is formed by hydrogen ... The atmosphere in question is low, its level very uneven and broken: often it does not rise above the projections of the photosphere, but the remarkable phenomenon is that it forms a continuous whole with the prominences, the composition of which is identical and which appear to be simply raised portions of it, projected and often detached in isolated clouds (*Comptes rendus hebdomadaires de l'Académie des sciences* 68 (1869): 181).

It is likely that Janssen discovered the helium D3 line, although it appears that he never fully understood this discovery, or at least never mentions it in any of his reports.

During the Franco-Prussian war, Janssen had decided to observe the eclipse of 22 December 1870 in Algeria. But how was he able to leave Paris which was then under siege? There was only one solution: the aerial route. A balloon, the Volta, was placed at his disposal and Janssen left Paris with an assistant on 2 December.

Janssen thought that 'the photographic plate is the retina of the scientist' (*L'astronomie* 2 (1883): 128). He was one of the first to understand that a photograph can do more than record what the eye perceives: 'I realized that photography ought to have a distinct advantage over optical observation in bringing out effect and relationships of light that are imperceptible to sight' (*Association française pour l'avancement des sciences*). The technique of short exposures led him in 1873 to design a device of historical interest: the 'photographic revolver', which can be considered as the precursor of cinematographic apparatus.

In 1874, the French government decided to establish an observatory for physical astronomy at Meudon. The most famous of Janssen's projects at Meudon was the atlas of solar photographs. Composed of a selection of exposures made between 1876 and 1903, it summarized the history of the surface of the sun during these years. It was not possible to make all the solar observations at Meudon. Janssen was well aware of the advantages of making observation at high altitudes. He went in October 1888 to the Mont Blanc massif to the refuge of the Grands Mulets at an altitude of 3,000 meters. His age and his lameness did not allow him to make the climb on foot, especially at that season. Thus he invented a conveyance to be borne by porters. The ascent, which lasted thirteen hours, was as exhausting for Janssen as for his porters. But the instruments were installed immediately, and the observations were sufficient to provide a solution to the problem under study. The dark rays were either nonexistent or so weak that it could be deduced that they would not exist for an observer at the limit of the terrestrial atmosphere.

Encouraged by this experiment, Janssen repeated it in 1890, this time working at the summit of Mont Blanc (4,800 meters). The measurements confirmed the earlier results. Despite the difficulties encountered, Janssen decided to erect an observatory there for conducting studies in physical astronomy, terrestrial physics, and meteorology. By July 1891, he had obtained the necessary funds and equipment, and two years later the observatory was completed. The initial construction was completed at Meudon, where a fifteen-ton building had been set up, which was then transported to Mont Blanc in pieces.

Although his observatory did not withstand the rigors of the weather, Janssen was widely admired for his energy and unfailing courage. He had acquired an international reputation early in his career. He was elected to the Academy of Sciences in 1873 and to the Bureau of Longitudes in 1875 and was also a member of major scientific organizations including the academies of Rome, Brussels, St. Petersburg, Edinburgh and in the United States.

He carried out his duties as director of the Meudon observatory until his death on 23 December 1907 which was the result of a pulmonary congestion.

In the words of Flammarion, 'He was 83 years old, and it is not quite elderly for the astronomic longevity'.

In light of his courage and persistence, it is not surprising that Janssen was able to accomplish so much that he undertook. As he himself wrote, 'There are very few difficulties that cannot be surmounted by a firm and a sufficiently thorough preparation'.

Acknowledgments

I would like to thank Mrs. Françoise Launay, assistant in the laboratory of Meudon, for helping me to find documents on Janssen's life.

Address for correspondence: Prof. Pierre Amalric, MD, Centre Médical Ophtalmologique, 6 rue Saint-Clair, F-81000 Albi, France.

Documenta Ophthalmologica **81**: 43–51, 1992.

John Cunningham Saunders (1773–1810):
His contribution to the surgery of congenital cataracts

NOEL S.C. RICE
London, England

Key words: History of ophthalmology, J.C. Saunders, congenital cataract

John Cunningham Saunders (Fig. 1), was born in Devonshire in 1773 and at the age of seventeen was apprenticed to a surgeon named John Hill in the town of Barnstaple, Devon. He served his apprenticeship for five years before moving to London where he studied at St. Thomas' Hospital and Guy's Medical School under Astley Cooper. He was subsequently appointed demonstrator of anatomy at St. Thomas' Hospital, succeeding Astley Cooper in that post. Because he had not been an apprentice at the Royal College of Surgeons, he was not eligible for an appointment to a London teaching hospital. However, he set up in practice and was the first regularly trained surgeon in Britain to devote himself exclusively to diseases of the eye and ear. In October 1804 he published a proposal to found a charitable institution for the cure of diseases of the eye and the ear. He was inspired to do so by a perception of an increase in eye disease in the country, a major contributory element in this being the number of cases of so-called Egyptian ophthalmia. This was a purulent conjunctivitis largely due to trachoma which had been contracted by troops serving in the Napoleonic campaign in Egypt. The charity was instituted and in March 1805 The London Dispensary for Curing Diseases of the Eye and Ear opened in Charterhouse Square (Fig. 2) with Saunders as its first surgeon. He soon recognised that his skill could be best served by limiting his practice to diseases of the eye and in 1808 he convinced the governors of the hospital of the wisdom of this action and they agreed to change the name of the hospital to The London Infirmary for Curing Diseases of the Eye. This institution subsequently became Moorfields Eye Hospital.

In a report to the committee of the charity in 1808 he wrote,

There is one point on which I must beg the indulgence of expatiating; I mean the adaptation of an operation on a cataract to the condition of childhood, by which I have successfully cured without a failure 14 persons born blind, some of them even in infancy, and it has just been performed on an infant only two months old, who is in a state of convalescence. As I reserve for another occasion the communication of the method which I pursue for the cure of very young children, I shall no further compare it

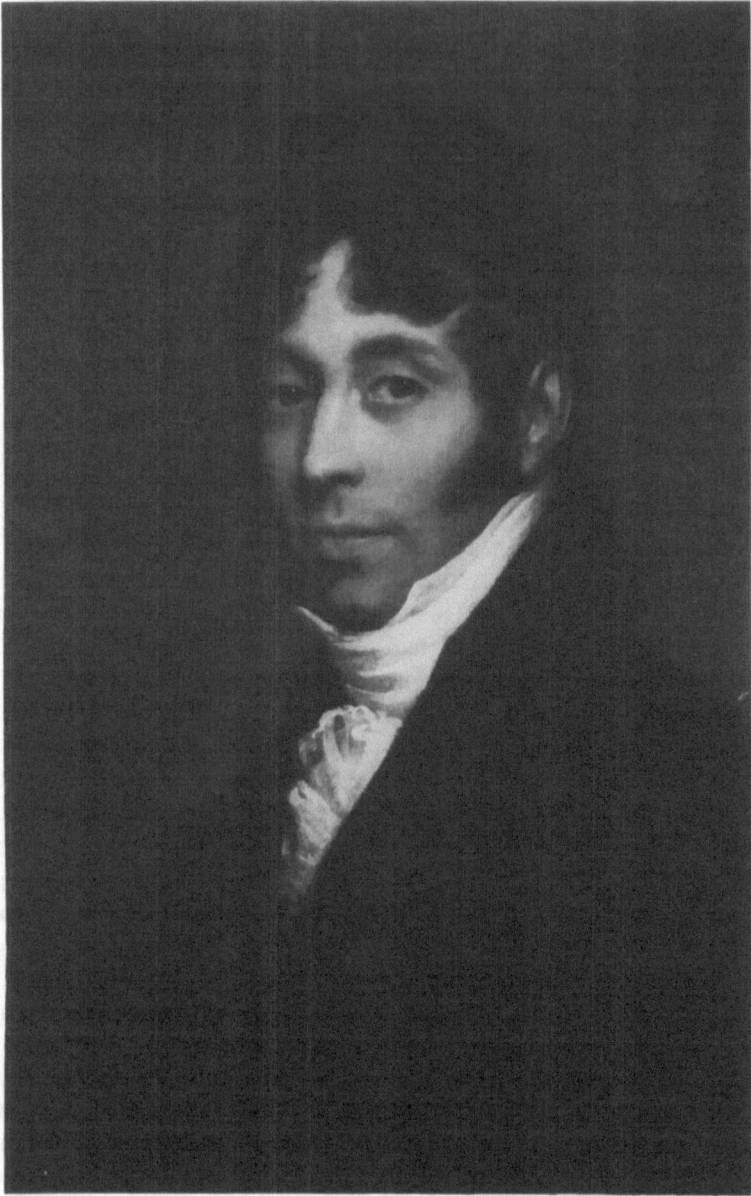

Fig. 1. John Cunningham Saunders (1773–1810). Portrait in the Board Room of Moorfields Eye Hospital.

with extraction, and by observing, that extraction is wholly inapplicable to children, or only fortuitously successful. Those who on all occasions adhere to this operation, and have never turned their thoughts towards the application of means more suitable to this tender age, have been

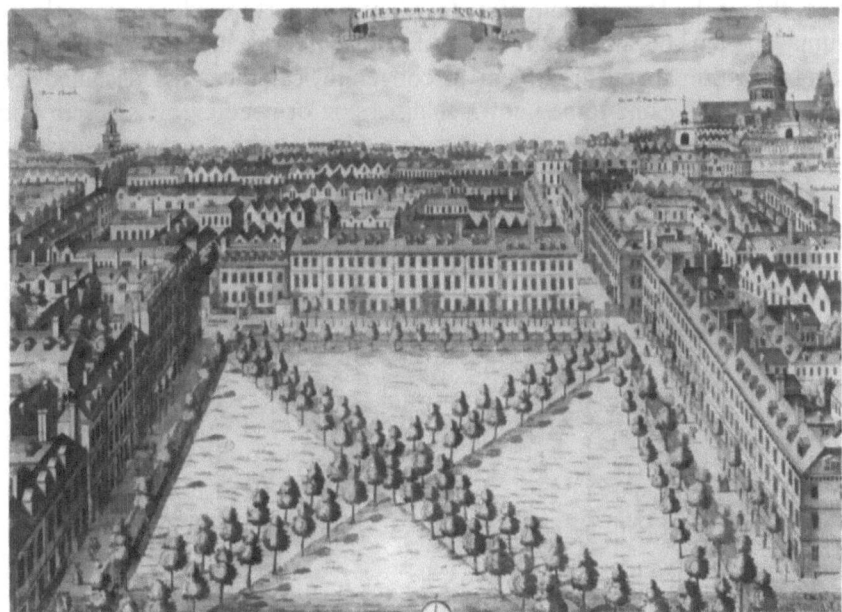

Fig. 2. View of Charterhouse Square, the site of the London Dispensary for curing diseases of the eye and ear.

obliged to wait until the patient has acquired sufficient reason to be tractable; otherwise when they have deviated from this conduct, the event has afforded little cause of self-congratulation. How great the advantage of an early cure, is a question of no difficult solution. Eyes originally affected with cataracts contract an unsteady and rolling motion, which remains after their removal, and retards, even when it does not ultimately prevent, the full benefit of the operation. A person cured at a late period cannot overcome this awkward habit by the utmost exertion of reason or the efforts at will but the actions of the infant are instinctive. Surrounding objects attract attention and the eye naturally follows them. The management of the eye is therefore readily acquired as vision rapidly improves and he will most probably be susceptible of education about the usual period. I am gentleman your obedient servant, J.C. Saunders.

At that time it was recognised that the available methods of treating cataracts in adults, extraction or couching, were inapplicable to young children, the results in Saunders' own words 'affording little cause for self-congratulation'; but he perceived that the current practice of delaying surgery for congenital cataracts until the age of ten or more years, even when technically satisfactory, gave very poor visual results; he associated this with the presence of nystagmus which he realized was an indicator of impaired visual development. He reasoned that if surgery could be carried out successfully on much younger children, the visual result should be better. It was already known from the observations of Percival Pott amongst others that if the lens capsule of a clear lens was perforated, for example by trauma, the lens became cataractous and subsequently absorbed. He applied this observation to the treatment of congenital cataracts and designed the operation which came to be known as discission or needling. His description of the techniques of surgery which he developed with great precision and

A

TREATISE

ON

SOME PRACTICAL POINTS

RELATING TO THE

DISEASES OF THE EYE;

BY THE LATE

JOHN CUNNINGHAM SAUNDERS,

DEMONSTRATOR OF ANATOMY AT SAINT THOMAS'S HOSPITAL,

𝔉ounder and 𝔖urgeon

OF THE

LONDON INFIRMARY FOR CURING DISEASES OF THE EYE.

———◆———

TO WHICH IS ADDED,

A SHORT ACCOUNT OF THE AUTHOR'S LIFE,

AND HIS METHOD OF

CURING THE CONGENITAL CATARACT,

BY HIS FRIEND AND COLLEAGUE,

J. R. FARRE, M. D.

THE WHOLE ILLUSTRATED BY COLOURED ENGRAVINGS.

———◆———

LONDON:

PRINTED FOR LONGMAN, HURST, REES, ORME, AND BROWN, PATERNOSTER-ROW; AND E. COX, ST. THOMAS'S STREET, BOROUGH.

———

1811.

Fig. 3. Title page of Saunders' *Treatise*.

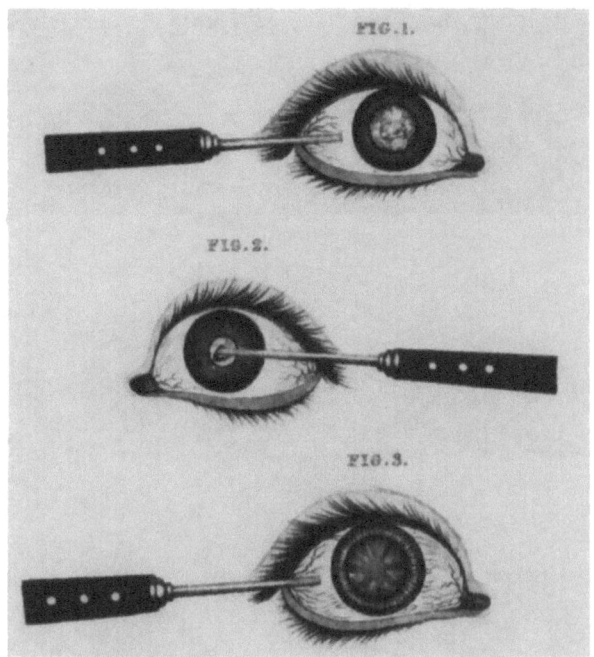

Fig. 4. Saunders techniques for discission.

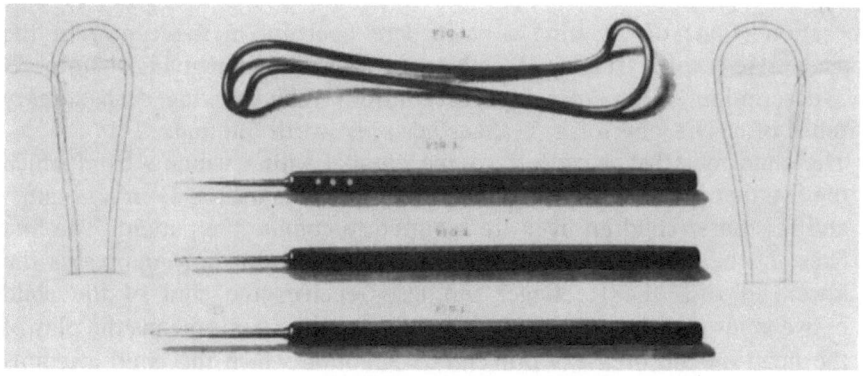

Fig. 5. Saunders' instruments for discission (Plate VIII of *Treatise*).

detail were published posthumously in *A treatise on some practical points relating to the diseases of the eye* (Figs. 3–6). This treatise was edited by his friend and colleague at Moorfields, J.R. Farre. Essentially he performed multiple needlings until the lens was absorbed and subsequently needled the remaining capsule with the aim 'ultimately to fulfill the intention of the

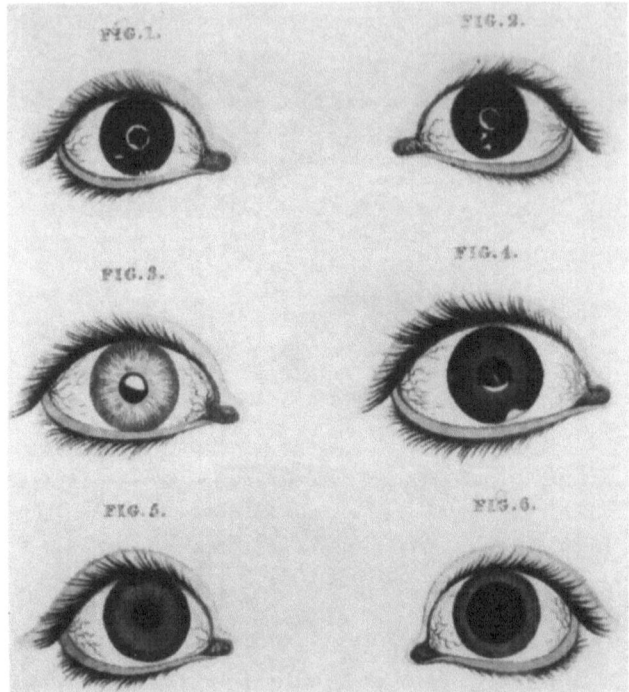

Fig. 6. Postoperative appearances of some eyes treated by Saunders for congenital cataract.

operation (that) of effecting a permanent aperture in the centre of the capsule'. He records treating 60 children and succeeded in giving sight to 52. His description of the measures to control a child having such surgery without of course any form of anaesthesia, is worth quoting:

The child must be placed on a table parallel with a window from which the eye that is to be submitted to the operation is farthest. Four assistants, and in stouter children five, are required to confine the patient. The first fixes the head with reversed hands, the second not only depresses the lower lid with the forefinger but also receives the chin of the child between his thumb and forefinger as in a crutch. By this means the play of the head on the breast is prevented, a motion which the child attempts incessantly and which will very much embarrass the surgeon. The third assistant confines the upper extremities in the body, the fourth the lower extremities. The surgeon seated on a high chair behind the patient and taking a Pellier's elevator in his left hand and the author's needle in his right if he is about to operate on the right eye, or the speculum in his right hand and the needle in his left if the operation is to be performed on the left eye, proceeds.

The needle he designed for this operation bears his name and is still familiar to many of us. Indeed the operation he designed remained the standard

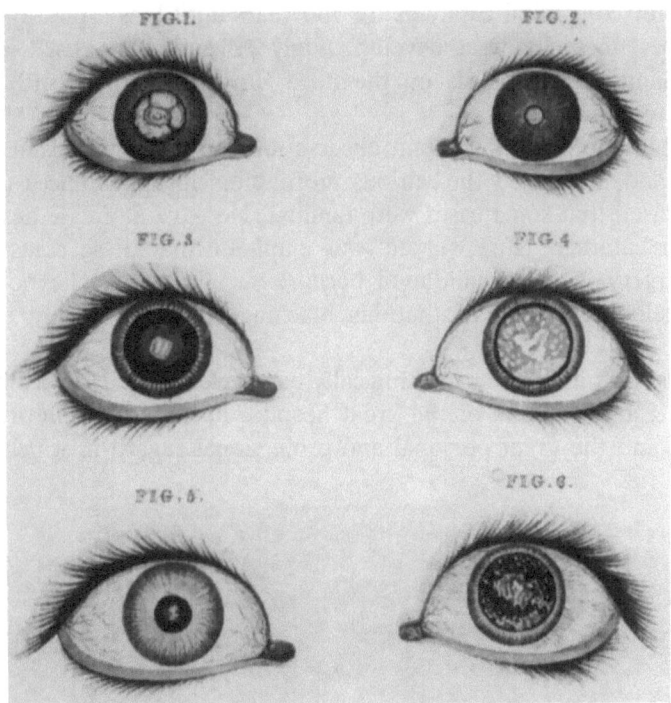

Fig. 7. Various morphological appearances of congenital cataracts described by Saunders.

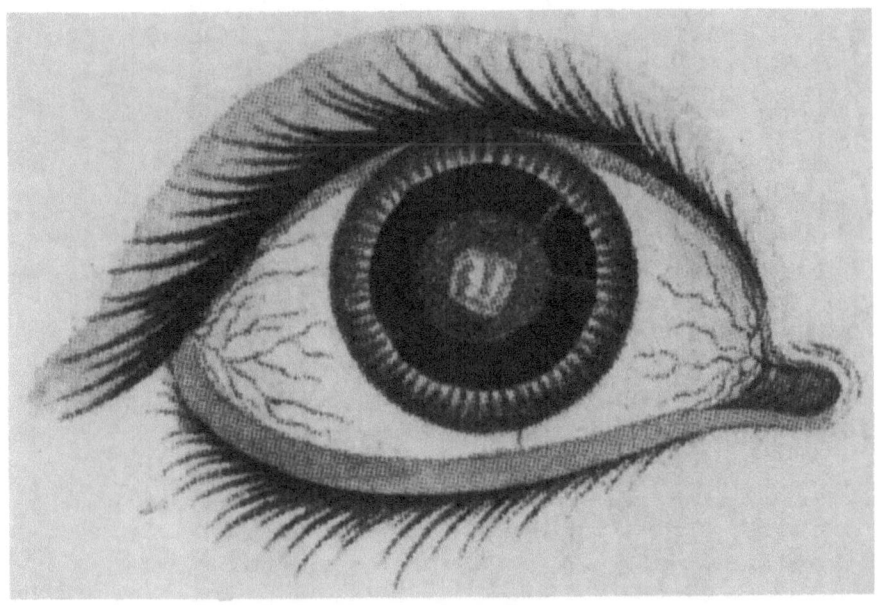

Fig. 8. Detail (part 3) from Fig. 7 illustrating lamellar cataract.

treatment for congenital cataracts for 150 years until lens aspiration and its subsequent refinements were developed only 25 years or so ago. One has to say that Saunders' emphasis on the need for early surgery still requires repetition today.

Saunders made other important observations on congenital cataracts. He described and illustrated the various morphological appearances (Fig. 7), and recognised that some cases were familial. He gave a precise description of lamellar cataracts (Fig. 8), and was emphatic that these cases did not require surgery in early childhood because such cataracts did not impair visual development. Would that his teaching were universally observed today!

Saunders died in 1810 at the tragically early age of 36. He was mourned by the staff and patients of the great hospital he founded only five years previously and the great personal and professional regard in which he was

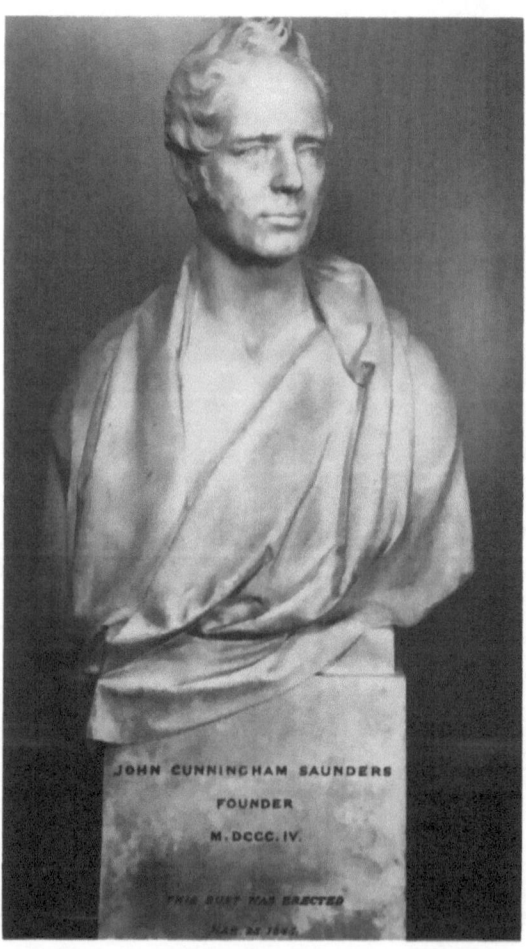

Fig. 9. Bust of Saunders in the Board Room of Moorfields Eye Hospital.

held is indicated by the resolutions which were moved at meetings of the general committee of the hospital and the Board of Governors.

That the committee unfailingly lament the irreparable loss this charity and society at large has sustained by the death of J.C. Saunders Esq., late surgeon to this infirmary. That this committee have ever recognised in Mr. Saunders the union of the most singular simplicity of character and the highest order of talents. That his humanity in the treatment of the poor objects of this charity has only been equalled by the extraordinary skill he has applied to their relief. That the adaptation of an operation to the cure of children born blind with cataract afforded the assurance of further extensive benefit to society and entitled him to rank as a benefactor to mankind.

It was further resolved that the treatise which Saunders had been preparing for publication should be published at the expense of the hospital to the benefit of his widow. Furthermore that a portrait and bust of Saunders (Fig. 9), should be obtained and placed in the Committee Room. Both the portrait and the bust referred to remain in the Board Room at Moorfields Eye Hospital to this day.

Acknowledgements

Figs. 1, 2, and 9 are reproduced by kind permission of the Governors of Moorfields Eye Hospital. Figs. 3 to 8 (drawings by H. Thomson, engraved by J. Stewart) are taken from Saunders' Treatise. I am indebted to Professor Barry Jay for drawing my attention to the contribution made by Saunders to the surgery of congenital cataracts.

Address for correspondence: Dr. Noel S.C. Rice, 25 Wimpole Street, London W1M 7AD, England.

Documenta Ophthalmologica **81**: 53–58, 1992.
© 1992 *Kluwer Academic Publishers.*

Thomas Hall Shastid (1866–1947):
America's forgotten historian of ophthalmology

FRANK W. NEWELL

Department of Ophthalmology and Visual Science, The University of Chicago

Key words: History of ophthalmology, T.H. Shastid

The *American Encyclopedia of Ophthalmology* [1] was edited by Casey A. Wood (1856–1942), of Chicago, and was published in 18 volumes between 1913 and 1921. It encompassed the whole of ophthalmology and more than 100 different ophthalmologists wrote various sections. Thomas Hall Shastid (1866–1947) was a major author and his contributions were exceeded only by those of Wood. Shastid provided over 500,000 words in 3,000 biographies, a first-class 375-page history of ophthalmology, a 150-page section on legal relations in ophthalmology (published in 1916 as a separate book [2]), and other sections describing a variety of topics. Shastid probably wrote somewhat more than ten percent of the 18 volumes. Today his biographies and history are nearly the sole items of lasting value in the Encyclopedia. Between 1918 and 1926 he wrote a number of biographies in the *American Journal of Ophthalmology*, which named him a collaborator in 1918, when the third series originated with Edward Jackson as editor. Between 1923 and 1926 he wrote three novels [3–5]. After 1925 Shastid stopped writing biographies for the *American Journal of Ophthalmology* and was no longer listed on the editorial board as a collaborator. He wrote two lengthy autobiographies [6, 7], a number of essays and books condemning war [8–10], abbreviated histories of ophthalmology, and a number of popular articles on ophthalmic topics [11–14].

Shastid was born in 1866, in Pittsfield, a farming community in the southern portion of the midwestern state of Illinois. He was the son of a physician. Pittsfield is a few miles from New Salem, where Abraham Lincoln clerked in a store as a youth and Lincoln and his friends were well known to the Shastid family [15]. John Nicolay, editor of the Pittsfield newspaper and subsequently President Lincoln's private secretary, was a boyhood friend of Shastid's father. John Milton Hay, a boyhood friend of Shastid, was a reporter for the Pittsfield newspaper and subsequently became a diplomat, United States Secretary of State, and co-author with Nicolay of the 10 volume biography of Lincoln [16].

Shastid's childhood was uneventful. His small stature led him to learn to box and this skill led to a fistfight with a classmate when he was a senior at Eureka College (from which President Ronald Reagan graduated in 1932).

Shastid's five classmates in the senior class voted that he not be permitted to graduate and that he be demoted to the junior class. This injustice so rankled him that thereafter he never mentioned Eureka College by name. In both of his autobiographies he refers to it as Inventi College. (He does, however, list it in his biography in *Who's Who in America*.) Shastid believed that it was not only the fistfight that upset his teachers and classmates, but also his heretical belief that germs caused disease and not possession by demons. Despite his complaints concerning Eureka College, Shastid was proficient in French, German, Greek, and Latin. He later added Arabic and a smattering of other languages to Choctaw, an American Indian language that he learned as a child.

Rather than return to Eureka College, Shastid, at 20 years of age, enrolled in the College of Physicians and Surgeons of Columbia University in 1886. Immediately after his arrival in New York City, Cornelius Rea Agnew, MD, professor of ophthalmology at the College, provided him with spectacles that relieved his ocular symptoms and possibly swayed him toward specializing in ophthalmology. He tells of the visit to Agnew in both the Encyclopedia and his autobiography. In 1887 the school moved to 59th Street and 10th Avenue, and increased its requirements for the MD degree from two years to three years. Shastid then transferred to the University of Vermont from which he received the M.D. degree with honors in 1888.

He did not return to Pittsfield, but travelled at once to Vienna where he concentrated on ophthalmology. After one year's study in Vienna Shastid joined his father in general practice in Pittsfield. He complained of the unwillingness of general practitioners to refer patients to specialists because they considered cultivation of a speciality a form of advertising or a sign of inability to practice all phases of medicine. Conversely, Pittsfield was far too small to require an ophthalmologist-otologist, and his fellow practitioners may have regarded Shastid as a competitor because he also saw patients in general practice.

In February 1892, after less than three years of practice with his father, Shastid travelled to Boston to apply for admission to the junior class of Harvard College. His application was rejected and he appealed to President Charles Eliot, who roared with laughter after Shastid described the Eureka College incident. Eliot intervened with the committee on admissions and Shastid received the Bachelor of Arts degree, cum laude, in 1893.

Shastid then practiced in several Illinois villages and towns with small professional success. In 1898 his practice in Galesburg, Illinois was unrewarding and his health was failing because of chronic appendicitis (his diagnosis). He went to a spa at Battle Creek, Michigan, but his health failed to improve. He consulted the professor of surgery at the University of Michigan (Charles B. De Nancrede, AM, MD, LLD) who promised a cure within two years. Shastid's health improved, but there is no mention in either of his autobiographies to indicate that the appendix was ever removed. In later years he attributed a chronic femoral phlebitis to the earlier

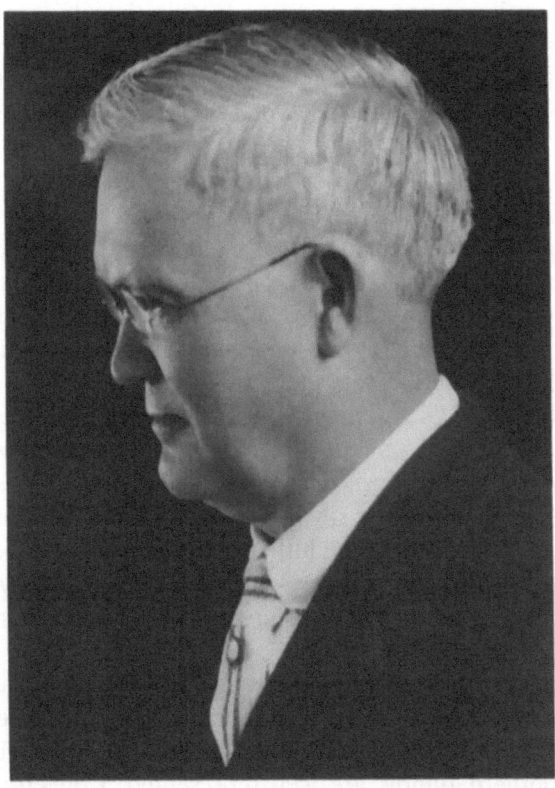

Fig. 1. Thomas Hall Shastid, about 1935, in a picture that he described as his favorite (from *My Second Life*, Ann Arbor, MI: G. Wahr, 1944).

appendicitis. There is no mention of an appendectomy in either of his autobiographies.

Shastid moved to Ann Arbor and enrolled in the College of Arts and Sciences and the Law School of the University of Michigan. He received a Master of Arts degree in 1901 and the Bachelor of Law degree in 1902. He served on the University Law Review and was admitted to the Michigan Bar and the federal courts. He subsequently wrote much about malpractice and the relationships of law and medicine, but never practiced law.

Shastid returned to Illinois and practiced in Fairfield and Harrisburg – towns too small to support an ophthalmologist-otologist. He eventually moved to Marion, in southern Illinois. While there he was named (1907) professor of the history of medicine at the American Medical College in St. Louis, a post to which he commuted until 1912. Thereafter, he was an honorary professor.

In July 1913, Shastid started practice with a clinic group in Duluth, Minnesota, but lived in nearby Superior, Wisconsin for the next eight years. Immediately after the move he was bedridden for six months and mortgaged his house to pay living expenses. Prior to this time he seemed to have adequate funds to pay for an extensive education and a series of failing professional endeavors. Shastid served as editorial secretary for the *Ophthalmic Record*, edited by Casey A. Wood, MD, from May until December 1913 [17].

In about 1911, Shastid first met with Casey Wood, who practiced in Chicago, and began his work on the *American Encyclopedia of Ophthalmology*. During subsequent years he travelled from Chicago, to Cleveland, to New York, vainly seeking a focus of infection that was causing a chronic femoral phlebitis. Although a number of specialists assured him he did not have sinus disease, he finally found a specialist in Duluth who operated on his sinuses and cured him.

Unfortunately, Shastid's autobiographies contain little detailed mention of the 27 years he practiced in Duluth. During this time, he wrote several novels, lectured widely, and practiced successfully. He was instrumental in the adoption of the compulsory silver nitrate law for newborns in the state of Wisconsin. Shastid died in Duluth on 15 February 1947. His library consisting of some 15,000 volumes, that dealt with slavery, witchcraft, medicine, literature, philosophy, music, and theology, each systematically indexed, was auctioned [18].

The *Encyclopedia of Ophthalmology* was his major work and its editor Casey Wood, was the major professional figure in his life. The biographies vary in quality. Shastid included many homeopathic practitioners, and specialists in southern Illinois are well represented. Conversely, the biographies each contain the essential data concerning the individual and provides the interested reader with a far easier source of biographic information than Hirschberg. He wrote a number of first-class biographies and the historian would do well to consult Shastid before undertaking additional research. In his biographies Shastid writes entertainingly of the unwillingness of the families of deceased practitioners to provide biographic information for fear it would be unethical or alternatively, that they would be charged for the books.

Volume 5 of the Encyclopedia contains a reference in which Shastid credits Hirschberg as a biographic source. Subsequently, Hirschberg credits Shastid in footnotes as a source of his biographies of nine practitioners.

The section on legal relations in ophthalmology, some 150 pages, reflects Shastid's legal training. It was the basis for many monographs on related topics, including sections in Casey Wood's *System of Ophthalmic Operations* [19] and Ball's *Modern Ophthalmology* [20].

Shastid was in Vienna on 31 January 1889, when the Austrian Crown Prince Rudolf and the Baroness Versera were found dead at Mayerling. It led Shastid to mistrust forever every national ruler whom he believed to be either mentally defective or psychopathic. It was the beginning of a lifelong crusade to have the people, not their rulers, declare war. The Spanish-American War further aroused the pacifist in him, and thereafter Shastid strongly opposed war and believed that citizens would never approve entry in a war. His writings on the topic are among his best. With no written evidence, I believe that his many writings concerning peace were the basis for the 1922 award of the honorary Doctor of Science degree by the University of Wisconsin (the secretary of faculties advises me that the citation has been lost). Conversely, the establishment of the silver nitrate law to prevent ophthalmia neonatorum may have been the reason.

Shastid's several novels are long and difficult reading. I found myself in full agreement with the review by the Anglican Archbishop of Sault Ste. Marie, Michigan, George Algoma, which was published in the front matter of the novel, 'Duke of Duluth', 'I have read the volume (Simon of Cyrene) with interest. It is certainly a remarkable book'. Shastid devotes several pages of the autobiographies to denouncing editors and book reviewers, although he apparently considered the remarks of the Archbishop as laudatory.

The autobiographies, *Tramping to Failure* (1937, 504 pages), and *My Second Life* (1944, 1,174 pages), are not conventional. Each consists of a series of vignettes, some of which are repeated in *My Second Life*. In a sense, Shastid's novels and autobiographies detract from his historical contributions, for they are by no means as well done.

Shastid published much on clinical ophthalmology and in his early days, on clinical otology, but there is little of permanent value. His autobiographies reflect a firm belief in focal infection as a cause of distant inflammation. Some of his medical writings were personally printed and distributed. He lectured widely to professional and lay groups on the theory of light, medical history, comparative anatomy, war and peace, and led a busy professional life. Thanks mainly to Casey Wood, he received national and international honors, but today he is little remembered, either as a popular author or as a physician.

References

1. Wood CA, ed: The American Encyclopedia and Dictionary of Ophthalmology, 18 vols. Chicago: Cleveland Press, 1913–1921.
2. Shastid TH: Ophthalmic Jurisprudence. Chicago: Cleveland Press, 1916.
3. Shastid TH: Simon of Cyrene, Dimachaerus Spelendius; or The Story of a Man's (and A Nation's) Soul. Ann Arbor, MI: G Wahr, 1923.
4. Shastid TH: Who Should Command the Heart? A Starlight Tale. Ann Arbor, MI: G Wahr, 1924.
5. Shastid TH: The Duke of Duluth, 2 vols. Ann Arbor, MI: G Wahr, 1926.
6. Shastid TH: Tramping to Failure. Ann Arbor, MI: G Wahr, 1937.
7. Shastid TH: My Second Life. Ann Arbor, MI: G Wahr, 1944.
8. Shastid TH: Give the People Their Own War Power. Ann Arbor, MI: G Wahr, 1927.
9. Shastid TH: The Only Way. Duluth, MN: Conepus, 1926, 2nd ed.
10. Shastid TH: How to Stop War-time Profiteering. Ann Arbor, MI: G Wahr, 1937, 2nd ed.

11. Shastid TH: Our Own and Our Cousins' Eyes. Southbridge, MA: American Optical Co, 1926.
12. Shastid TH: An Outline History of Ophthalmology. Southbridge, MA: American Optical Co, 1927.
13. Shastid TH: Light, The Raw Material of Vision. Ann Arbor, MI: G Wahr, 1936.
14. Shastid TH: Eyes that a sportsman should have. Field and Stream 1926, 31: 12.
15. Shastid TH: My father knew Lincoln. Nation 1929, 60: 824.
16. Nicolay JG, Hay J: Abraham Lincoln: A History, 10 vols. New York: The Century, 1890.
17. Wood CA: Veleditory. Ophthalmic Record 1917, 26: 499.
18. Hilding AC: Obituary Tomas Hall Shastid (1866–1947). Am J Ophthalmol 1947, 30: 1445–1446.
19. Shastid TH: The forensic relations in ophthalmic surgery, Vol 1, pp. 43–179, in Wood CA, ed: A system of Ophthalmic Operations, 2 vols. Chicago: Cleveland Press, 1911.
20. Shastid TH: The legal relations in ophthalmology, Vol 2, pp. 1343–1347, in Ball JM, ed: Modern Ophthalmoloyg, 2 vols. Philadelphia, CA: Davis, 1925, 5th ed.

Address for correspondence: Frank W. Newell, MD, Department of Ophthalmology and Visual Science, The University of Chicago, 937 East 57th Street, Chicago, IL 60637, USA.

Documenta Ophthalmologica **81**: 59–73, 1992.

William R. Wilde (1815–1876) in Vienna

FREDERICK C. BLODI

Department of Ophthalmology, University of Iowa

Key words: History of ophthalmology, William Wilde

William R. Wilde was born 1815 in a small hamlet in Connaught, the most western part of Ireland. His father was English and a practicing physician while his mother was Irish. Numerous biographies describe his life [1], and an extensive obituary summarizes his achievement [2].

He began his medical education 1832 in Dublin as an apprentice to the celebrated Abraham Colles. He then became a resident pupil in Dr. Steevens' hospital to which at that period the flourishing Park Street Medical School was attached. He remained there for four years and worked with James Graves and William Stokes. Corpses for autopsy were obtained from resurrectionists (body snatcher). In 1832 he weathered – like everyone else in Ireland – a cholera epidemic. In 1837 he obtained his diploma of licentiate from the Royal College of Surgeons in Ireland (Fig. 1).

Shortly afterwards he was recommended by Sir Henry Marsh and Dr. Robert Graves (Fig. 2) to take charge of a patient who was sailing in his own yacht, the 'Crusades', to the Mediterranean. Wilde spent nine months

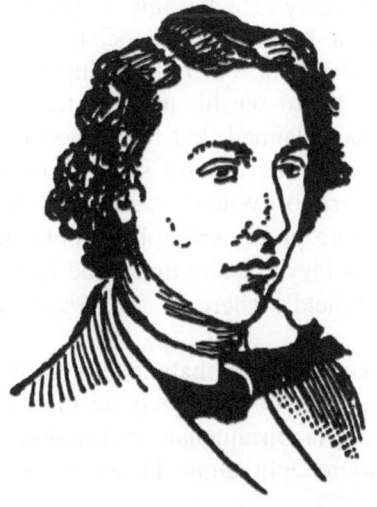

Fig. 1. William R. Wilde in 1837.

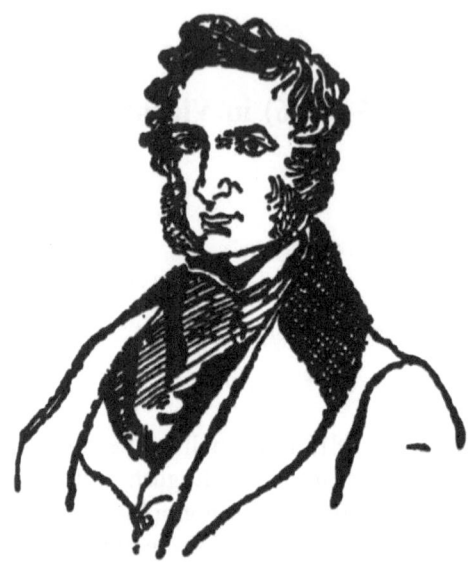

Fig. 2. Robert Graves, Wilde's teacher, also studied in Vienna.

there during which he saw a great number of cities and countries. In 1837 he visited Madeira and Teneriffe. The boat then sailed to Algeria, Alexandria and Cairo. Wilde saw many cases of trachoma in patients who were surrounded by starvation, filth and degradation. This apparently aroused his interest in ophthalmology. From Egypt they sailed to Rhodes and Palestine. A narrative of this voyage was published in 1840 [3]. This book became quite a success and revealed Wilde's keen interest in nature, science, scenery, topography, antiquities, folklore, etc.

In 1838 Wilde returned to Dublin and became a general practitioner who also performed minor surgery. He became a member of the Royal Irish Academy (Fig. 3) and of the British Association. At that time he also performed biological studies, e.g. on the suckling of whales.

Wilde had to travel a lot to see his many patients. He became quite a womanizer and G.B. Shaw claimed that he wanted to establish a family in every Irish hamlet. One of his natural sons apparently was Dr. Henry Wilson (an abbreviated form of 'Wilde's son'), 1838–1878, who was Wilde's assistant and then became a prominent ophthalmologist in Dublin (Fig. 4). He had studied ophthalmology in Cairo under the Frenchman Clot and then spent six months at Moorfield's where he was associated with William Farr and Sir James Clark.

Wilde decided to specialize in ophthalmic and aural surgery. He devoted the next three years studying these subjects on the continent, especially in Vienna. In 1839 he went via Birmingham to London, where he worked at Moorfield's Royal London Ophthalmic Hospital, mainly with Tyrell and Dalrymple.

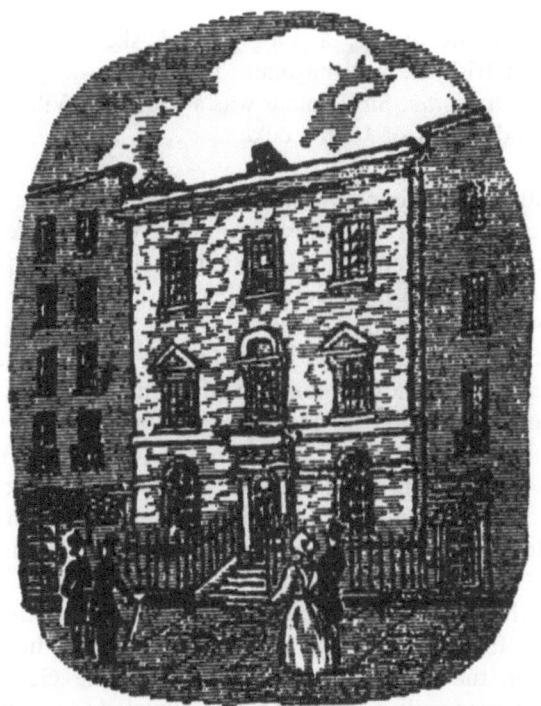

Fig. 3. The old Royal Irish Academy house on Grafton Street.

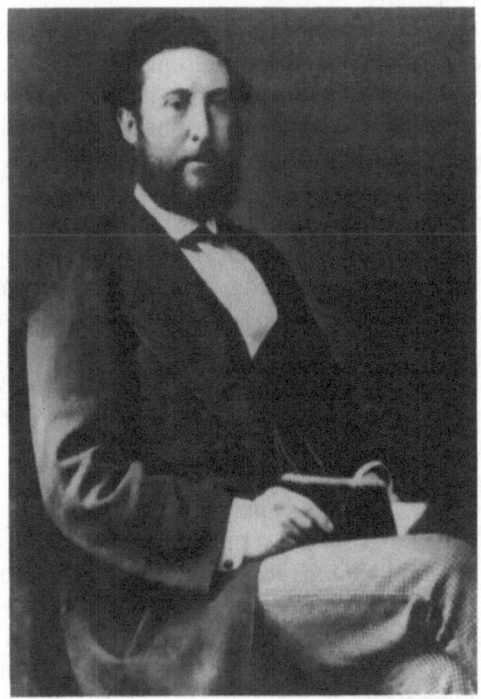

Fig. 4. Dr. Henry Wilson (Wilde's natural son), photograph in the Royal Eye and Ear Hospital, Dublin.

During that time he wrote a biographical sketch on Sir Thomas Molyneux, the first Irish medical baronet. The paper was published in the *Dublin University Magazine*. Sir Thomas was a cousin of William Molyneux, the philosopher and friend of John Locke.

Wilde spent 1840/41 in Vienna where he became a private pupil of the celebrated Professor Jaeger. On his return he wrote a report on the political, social and medical conditions in Biedermeier Vienna [4]. The book has recently been translated into German [5]. It was favorably reviewed in the *Dublin Journal of Medical Science* (23: 474, 1843). The anonymous reviewer calls it 'an invaluable boon conferred upon us, reflecting the highest credit upon the author's industry and talent' (Fig. 5).

This monograph is dedicated to Dr. Friedrich Jaeger, Professor of Ophthalmology at the Josephinum in Vienna and to Robert J. Graves, M.D., Queen's Professor, Institute of Medicine, School of Physic in Dublin, Ireland, who had several decades earlier also spent some time in Vienna studying ophthalmology. Wilde signs as friend and pupil in thankful recognition.

In the preface the author first points out under which circumstances this book was written. In the years 1840 and 1841, he visited the most famous medical schools on the continent, mainly those of the German-speaking states. He wanted especially to augment his knowledge in ophthalmology and otology. Vienna had such a high reputation in this area that he spent most of his time in that city.

Before leaving Ireland, Wilde found that there was no real guide or informational book available describing present day Austria. Certainly none that was concerned with medicine and public health in that country. In no other European country is it so difficult to obtain information of a general nature as in Austria. The censorship is severe. Wilde says about ophthalmology in Vienna:

For a century the Viennese school is in this specialty leading. Every ophthalmologist who wants to become a master of his specialty, should spend a few months in Vienna in order to attend the lectures and practical exercises of Jaeger and Rosas. In addition, he should seize the opportunity to participate in private courses on ophthalmic surgery.

The first chapter of his book deals with the structure of the Austrian empire, public school system, the variety of schools, elementary schools and kindergarten, the effects of the Austrian school system, and the obligatory instruction of religion.

Attending elementary school is mandatory. These schools are usually under the control of the parish priest, though non-catholic schools exist in some provinces. The middle education is dedicated either to the humanistic principles or to a more technical field. Higher education is offered at nine institutes in nine different cities. The University of Vienna is not only the oldest (founded 1365), but also the biggest Austrian institute of higher education. Modern medicine was introduced in Vienna by Boerhaave of

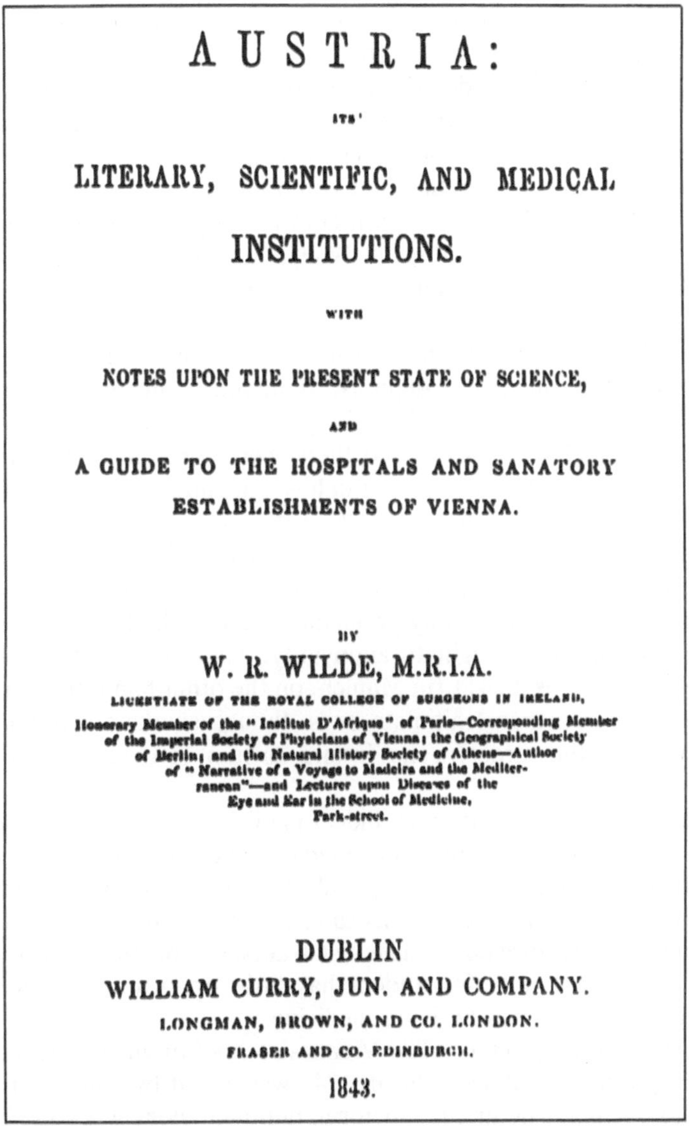

AUSTRIA:

ITS

LITERARY, SCIENTIFIC, AND MEDICAL

INSTITUTIONS.

WITH

NOTES UPON THE PRESENT STATE OF SCIENCE,

AND

A GUIDE TO THE HOSPITALS AND SANATORY
ESTABLISHMENTS OF VIENNA.

BY

W. R. WILDE, M.R.I.A.

LICENTIATE OF THE ROYAL COLLEGE OF SURGEONS IN IRELAND,
Honorary Member of the " Institut D'Afrique" of Paris—Corresponding Member
of the Imperial Society of Physicians of Vienna; the Geographical Society
of Berlin; and the Natural History Society of Athens—Author
of " Narrative of a Voyage to Madeira and the Mediterranean"—and Lecturer upon Diseases of the
Eye and Ear in the School of Medicine,
Park-street.

DUBLIN

WILLIAM CURRY, JUN. AND COMPANY.

LONGMAN, BROWN, AND CO. LONDON.

FRASER AND CO. EDINBURGH.

1843.

Fig. 5. Wilde's report on Austria (1843).

Leiden and then by his pupil, van Swieten, who was invited by the Empress
Maria Theresa to come to Vienna.

The second chapter of the book discusses surgery, pharmacy and pharmacology. The surgeons are also barbers who practice bloodletting, the use of
leeches, bandaging wounds and setting fractures. These surgeons have three
years of schooling, but cannot obtain the doctor degree. (They can be only
master of surgery.) They still have to have a barbershop attached to the

office though it can be managed by an assistant. Pharmacology and pharmacy are strictly regulated in Austria.

In chapter three Wilde describes Vienna with its sciences and arts. He regrets that there is no Austrian academy of science. Dancing and smoking are the most popular recreations. There is actually a mania for dancing without class distinction to the tunes of Lanner and Strauss and Wilde himself participated. Among his partners was the widowed daughter-in-law Ottilie of the great poet, Johann Wolfgang von Goethe. Literature is flourishing. There are also a number of scientific societies, museums and art galleries.

Chapter four deals with the Viennese General Hospital, which was founded 1784 by Emperor Joseph II. It admits indigent patients, treats patients for a fee, if they can afford it, and serves as a school for practical and clinical medicine. At that time there were three main buildings, the medical and surgical clinics, the lying-in hospital and the insane asylum. The hospital had 2,214 beds. There were 6 professors, 15 secondary physicians and 32 physicians in training. Strange is the custom that nurses, custodians and patients will kiss the hand of the professor when he enters the ward. The lying-in hospital admits any pregnant woman, whether she can pay or not. The women have a right to anonymity. The relation of legitimate to illegitimate children is 2.24:1 (in Munich, on the other hand, there are more illegitimate children than legitimate ones, though smokers and whores are not allowed on the street). The insane asylum is overcrowded and in desolate condition.

Chapter five is concerned with clinical medicine. The clinical teaching is one of the outstanding advantages of medical education in Austria. Instruction is mainly done at the bedside, while the professor and the physicians converse in Latin so that the patients cannot understand them. The teaching is exceptionally well organized. The disadvantages are: there are too many students per patient and the student has little opportunity to visit other clinical departments when he is on medicine.

Exemplary is the eye clinic. The Viennese school originated actually with the Italian physician Pallucci who in 1745 was called by van Swieten from Florence to Vienna. The first instructor in ophthalmology was Joseph Barth, who came from Malta, but was educated in Rome. He became professor of ophthalmology in Vienna in 1773. In 1776 he became personal physician to Emperor Joseph II. The actual founder of Viennese ophthalmology was Georg Joseph Beer, who in 1815 became chairman of the first university eye department in the world.

At the time of Barth, Joseph Mohrenheim and Franz Siegerist practiced ophthalmology in the city of Vienna. Other pupils of Barth were Joseph Adam Schmidt, later professor of surgery at the Josephinum Military Academy and Jacob Santerelli, who, for the first time, made the cataract incision at the upper limbus. Schmidt's successor is Friedrich Jaeger, who occupies the second chair of ophthalmology in Vienna.

At the moment, Professor Dr. Anton Edler von Rosas, a Hungarian physician, is chairman of the University Department of Ophthalmology, which has 150 beds. The professor lectures twice a week to the medical students. Ophthalmology is mandatory in the medical curriculum and each student has to pass an examination in practical ophthalmology. Anybody who wants to perform eye operations has to spend a fifth year of study and practice in the eye clinic. Rosas is a skillful surgeon and he invented his own cataract knife.

The new Viennese medical tradition is described in chapter six. Percussion and auscultation are an important aspect of the new medical education. The Institute for Pathologic Anatomy is directed by Professor Rokitansky, whose concept of dyscrasia dominates Austrian medicine. The Military Academy was founded 1785 by Emperor Joseph II and is now known as the 'Josephinum'. It contains nearly all branches of a medical school, but the most important and interesting aspect is the eye clinic of Professor Jaeger. It consists of two wards with 11 beds each. The students become military officers of the Austrian army and the patients are soldiers and their families.

Dr. Friedrich Jaeger, a former assistant of Beer, followed 1812 J.A. Schmidt as professor of ophthalmology at the Josephinum. He has become a famous surgeon and his private courses are one of the greatest medical attractions of the city of Vienna. Jaeger is the son-in-law of Beer and inherited the latter's library and collection of specimens and instruments.

In the Josephinum German is the official language.

Senile cataract and amblyopia are quite frequently seen in Vienna and the same holds for arthritic ocular changes, especially arthritic iritis. Syphilitic iritis is much rarer than in other countries, especially England. During the hot season, eye inflammations are here more frequent than in Ireland. In some cases, especially in soldiers, there is early pus formation and even an Egyptian ophthalmia may develop. The pannus is treated with the inoculation of ocular blennorrheic material, following the reports by D.F. Piringer in Graz. Jaeger apparently initiated this treatment 30 years earlier.

Jaeger published very little. Important is his monograph on Egyptian ophthalmia which caused havoc in the Austrian army. The cause of this affection is supposed to be a miasm which consists of impurities in the evaporations coming from the soil, from swamps, etc.

The most interesting and most fruitful aspect of ophthalmic education is the private course in ocular surgery which Professor Jaeger gives daily in his domicile from 2:00 to 3:00 p.m. The professor takes no more than six pupils at a time. At the present there were among the students Dr. Mackenzie of Glasgow, Mr. T. Wharton Jones of London and Dr. R. Dudgeon of Liverpool. A mannequin is used for practice. The patient sits on a stool in front of the surgeon and leans his head on the chest of an assistant who elevates the upper lid. Jaeger also practices couching and reclination. He may also perform a discission or dislaceration on the cataract. For the extraction he uses an incision at the upper limbus.

Unique is the anatomical museum of the Josephinum which consists of numerous wax models. Most of them were made by Tortona and Mascagni, two famous Florentine artists. In some rooms there are similar models of plants and of animals. Women cannot visit this museum.

Chapter thirteen deals with homeopathy, the status of the indigent population and the other Viennese hospitals. There is an excellent homeopathic hospital in a suburb. It is run by sisters. During the cholera epidemics a large number of patients were admitted and quite successfully treated by homeopathic methods.

There are in Vienna two public institutes for the blind, one for children and one for adults. There is also an institute for abandoned children established – like apparently everything else – by Joseph II. Veterinary medicine is taught in a separate college.

In the last chapter the author discusses public health issues in the Austrian empire, presenting statistics on mortality and morbidity frequencies.

Wilde describes in his book not only public health, medical practice and education, but makes also astute observations on the political and cultural scene. Austria was then an absolute monarchy and the chancellor, Prince Metternich, reigned without opposition. Wilde supported the aim of Baron Hammer-Purgstall, the famous orientalist, to establish an Austrian academy of science. Wilde admires the democratic attitude of the aristocracy, the relative wealth of the average citizen and merchant and the good life enjoyed by everybody. He deplores the absence of political freedom, the censorship, the general fear of innovation, emancipation and reform.

After Vienna he went to Munich and saw King Ludwig I, then to Prague where he visited Count Thun, later to Dresden where he conferred with the anatomist Carus and the physiologist Seiler. In Berlin he worked with the plastic surgeon Dieffenbach and assisted in a partial excision of a tongue which was supposed to cure stammering (to which a sharp-tongued friend remarked 'so does a hangman cure indigestion').

Returned to Ireland, he became Medical Census Commissioner in 1841. Wilde held this office until his death and the census of 1851, 1861 and 1871 all contained valuable work from his pen [6]. This work consumed a great deal of his effort and time. It included an analysis of all the pestilences, floods and catastrophes recorded in Ireland from the earliest period. In appreciation of his work as a medical commissioner he was knighted in 1864.

In 1841 he opened in his home (Fig. 6) a free dispensary for ophthalmic and aural diseases which in 1843 was replaced by a much larger public hospital, the St. Mark's Ophthalmic Hospital and Dispensary for Diseases of the Eye and Ear. This hospital published annual reports in which Wilde presented statistical data on the activities of the staff. In a report on 120 cases of strabismus operated within two years the success rate was 85%. There were a few instances of secondary exotropia and among them was G.B. Shaw's father. Wilde introduced atropine as a treatment of corneal ulcer and the cataract extraction into Ireland.

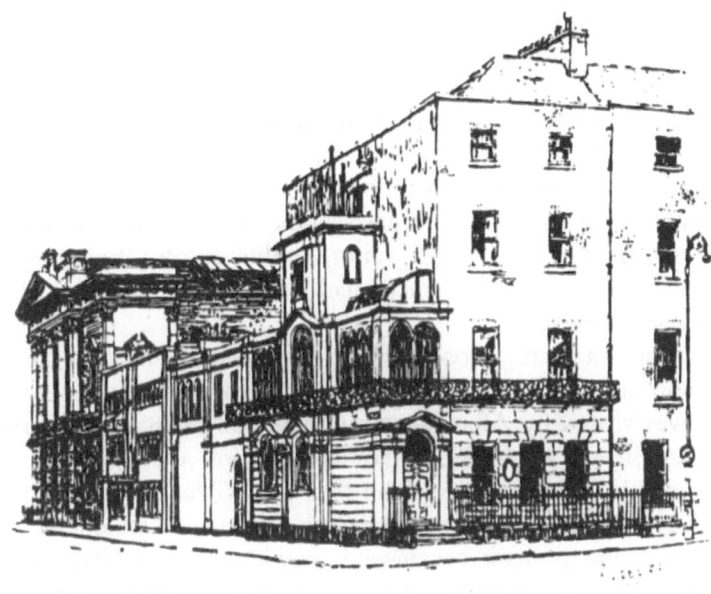

Fig. 6a. The Wilde residence, 1 Merrion Square (graphic by P. Liddy).

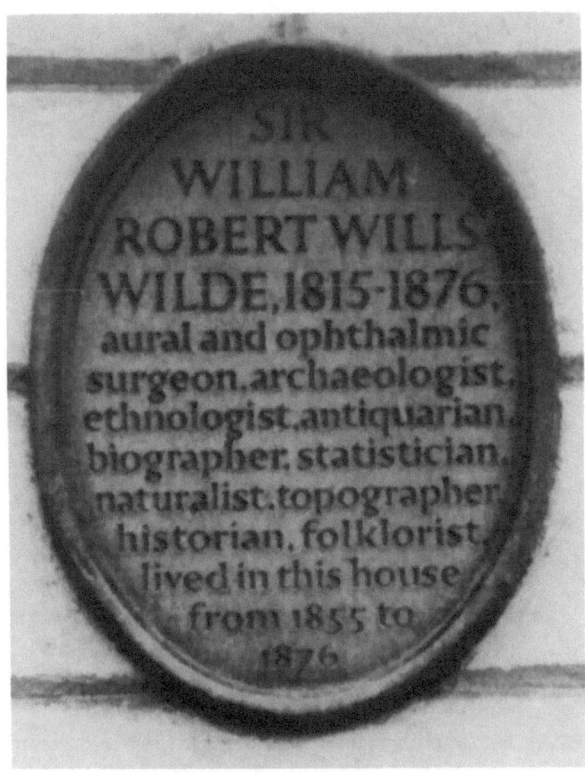

Fig. 6b. Plaque on Wilde's house.

In 1897, St. Mark's Hospital was amalgamated with the National Eye and Ear Infirmary and in this way the new Royal Victoria Eye and Ear Hospital was created.

Wilde participated in the battle against trachoma which at that time was quite prevalent in Ireland. He became a fellow of the Royal College of Surgeons of Ireland and in 1845 was appointed editor of the *Dublin Journal of Medical Science* (Fig. 7). This journal was the successor of *The Dublin Quarterly Journal of Medicine*, whose editor, Arthur Jacob [7] after whom the membrana Jacobi had been named, had been forced to resign. They remained enemies forever.

Wilde also wrote interesting books on the Irish scenery and topography, and made important contributions to the study of Irish antiquities.

In 1850 he was visited by Albrecht von Graefe and in 1851, he married Jane Francesca Elgee (1826–1896), the daughter of a clergyman. The ceremony was officiated by the Rev. John Maxwell Wilde, an elder brother of William. They had three children, a daughter who died in childhood, and two sons of whom the younger became the well-known poet Oscar Wilde (Fig. 8) [8]. His wife was a writer in her own right publishing under the pseudonym 'Speranza' (Fig. 9) [9].

The Wildes were certainly an eccentric couple. His reputation for lechery

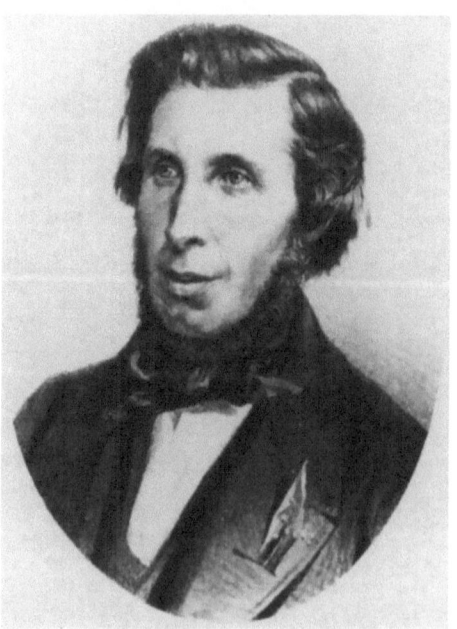

Fig. 7. William R. Wilde, lithograph by James Henry Lynch (from a daguerrotype by L. Gluckman, 1845).

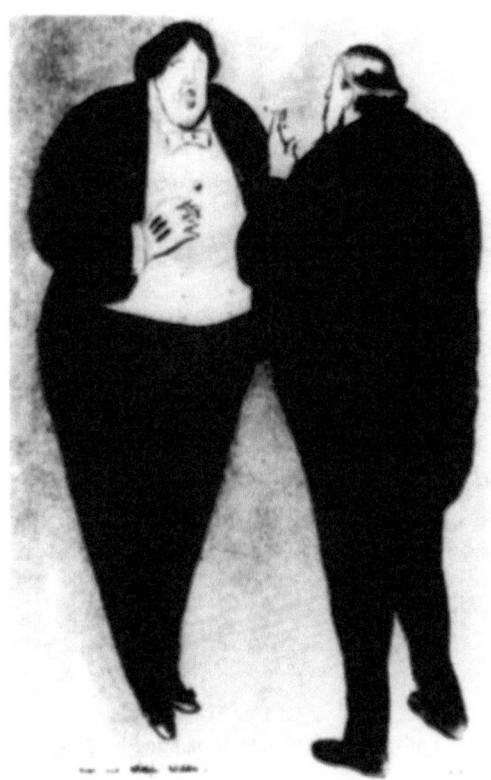

Fig. 8. Oscar Wilde (with white tie) and his brother, Willie, caricature by Sir Max Beerbohm (Humanities Research Center, University of Texas, Austin).

and her gigantism made them unusual and unorthodox parents (Fig. 10). They did not believe in cleanliness and attractiveness. Why does Wilde have black fingernails? Because he scratches himself, was the saying. Lady Wilde, on the other hand, 'with her paint and tinsel and tawdry, tragedy-queen get-up was a walking burlesque of motherhood. Her husband resembled a monkey, a miserable looking creature, apparently unshorn and unkept he looked as if he had been rolling in the dust'. [1d]. It is quite possible that this bizarre couple contributed to the homosexuality of their son, Oscar.

In his latter years he lost much of his wonderful energy and it was a matter of astonishment to his pupils that he never really mastered the ophthalmoscope. He was in the habit of sending his private patients to Mr. Henry Wilson to have the fundus examined. It was Wilson who had introduced the ophthalmoscope into Ireland. But Wilde continued to practice until he was over 60, making his daily rounds on horseback.

His later years were darkened by a libel case that impugned his honor. An unbalanced woman became his persecutor and filed suit against Lady Wilde because she had written a letter of condemnation to the young woman's

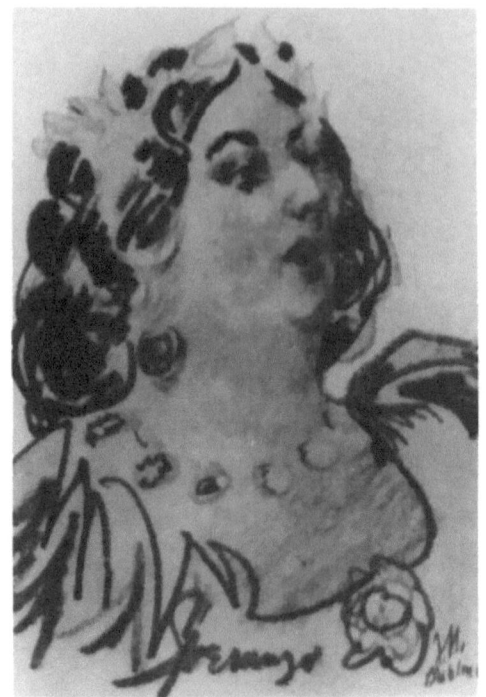

Fig. 9. Lady Wilde (Speranza), painting by J. Morosini.

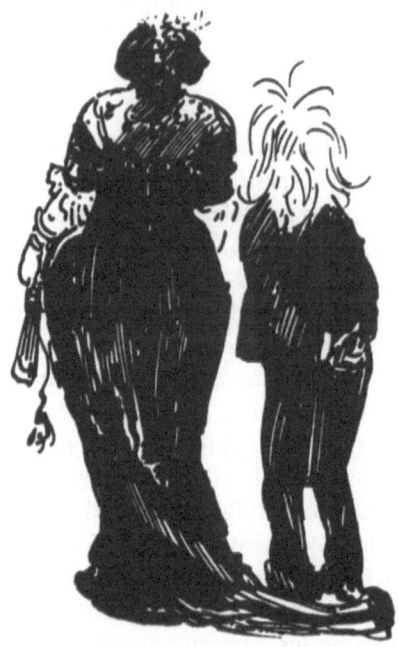

Fig. 10. Sir William and Lady Wilde, sketch by Harry Furniss.

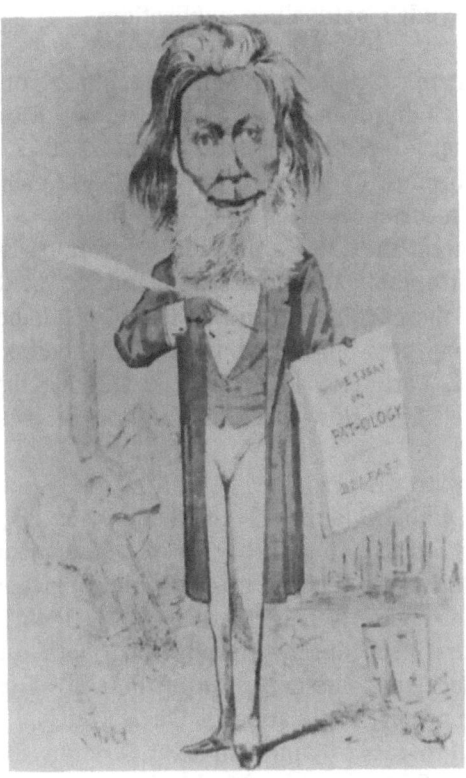

Fig. 11. A cartoon of Wilde as 'wild otologist', from the Irish magazine *Ireland's Eye.*

father. Lady Wilde was tried and fined a farthing. William Wilde never did appear in court, for which he was castigated by his enemy, Arthur Jacob [10]. He died peacefully 1876.

William Wilde emerges from all this as a man with wide interests and staggering accomplishments. He was a pioneer for Irish ophthalmology. His ophthalmic publications were solid and are listed in the appendix. He wrote many otologic papers and a book on this topic (*Practical Observations on Aural Surgery and the Nature and Treatment of Diseases of the Ear*, Philadelphia: Blanchard, 1853). He is regarded as one of the two or three most prominent British otologists of that century [11].

His work on the census contributed enormously to our knowledge on the demography of that country. He published valuable contributions to Irish history [12], geography [13], and anthropology [14]. He was truly a man for all seasons.

Speranza outlived him by twenty years. She emerges as a loving, indulgent mother and a loyal, courageous wife. It just so happened that their dazzling son, Oscar, outshone his parents by his life-style and his writings.

Appendix: List of Wilde's ophthalmic publications

1. On the Ophthalmic School of Vienna, Dublin J. of Medical Science (Exhibiting a Comprehensive Review of the Latest Discoveries in Medicine, Surgery and the Collateral Sciences) 20: 254, 1842.
2. Letter on Strabismus, ibidem 22: 163, 1842/43 [Against James Adams; Wilde saw no recurrences after his operations].
3. Observations upon the Causes and the Operations Recommended for the Cure of Entropium and Trichiasis, ibidem 25: 98, 1844 [lecture upon the diseases of the eye and ear in the School of Medicine Park-Street].
4. An Essay upon the Malformations and Congenital Diseases of the Organ of Sight, Part I [Read before the Dublin Obstetrical Society]: ibidem 27: 42, 1845 [Now also: Surgeon to St. Mark's Ophthalmic Hospital].
5. Part II, ibidem 28: 81, 1845.
6. Part III, The Dublin Quarterly J. of Medicine 6: 251, 1848.
7. The Editor's Preface: The history of periodic medical literature in Ireland, including notices of the medico-philosophical societies of Dublin, The Dublin Quarterly J. of Medicine 1: 1, 1846.
8. Some Particulars respecting Swift and Stella, with Engravings of their Crania (together with some notice on St. Patrick's Hospital), ibidem 7: 1, 1847 [Post-mortem examination of Dean Swift].
9. Report on the Progress of Ophthalmic Surgery for 1847, ibidem 8: 467, 1848 [Now only: Surgeon to St. Mark's Ophthalmic Hospital].
10. On the epidemic ophthalmia, London J. Medicine, 1851.
11. Report on the number, sex and condition of the blind, Med. Times and Gazette, 1862.

References

1. (a) Byrne, Patrick: The Wildes of Merrion Square. London/New York: Staples Press, 1953.
   (b) Lambert, E.: Mad With Much Heart – Life of the Parents of Oscar Wilde. London: Frederick Muller, 1967.
   (c) Somerville-Large, L.B.: The development of ophthalmology in Ireland. The Irish J. of Med. Sciences 1960; 411: 97.
   (d) Story, J.B.: Sir William Robert Wills Wilde. Brit. J. Ophth. 1918; 2: 65.
   (e) White, Terence de Vere: The Parents of Oscar Wilde. London: Hodder and Stoughton, 1967.
   (f) Wilson, Thomas George: Victorian Doctor – Being the Life of Sir William Wilde. New York: L.B. Fischer, 1946.
2. Obituary: Sir William Robert Wills Wilde. Med. Times and Gazette, 6 May 1876, p. 510.
3. Narration to a Voyage to Madeira, Teneriffe, and Along the Shores of the Mediterranean, including a Visit to Algiers, Egypt, Rhodes, Telmessus, Cyprus and Greece. With Observations on the Present State and Prospects of Egypt and Palestine, and on the Climate, Natural History, Antiquities, etc. of the Countries Visited. Dublin: W. Curry, Jr., 1840.
4. Austria and Its Literary, Scientific, and Medical Institutions; With Notes upon the Present

State of Science and a Guide to the Hospitals and Sanitary Establishments of Vienna. Dublin: W. Curry, Jr. and Co./London: Longman, Brown and Co. Edinburgh: Fraser and Co. 1843.

5. Montjoye, Irene (Ed.): Oscar Wildes Vater über Metternichs Österreich, Frankfurt am Main/Bern/New York/Paris: Verlag Peter Lang, 1989.

6. Ireland Census Office: Report of the Commissioners appointed to take the Census of Ireland for the Year 1841. Presented to both houses of parliament by command of Her Majesty. Printed by A. Thorn for H.M. Stationery Office, 1843.

7. Hirschberg, J.: The History of Ophthalmology, translated by F.C. Blodi, Vol. 8, p. 127. Bonn: J.P. Wayenborgh, 1988.

8. Ellermann, R.: Oscar Wilde. London: Hamish Hamilton, Inc., 1987.

9. Wyndham, Horace: Speranza, a biography of Lady Wilde. New York: Philosophical Library, 1951.

10. (a) Editorial, The Lancet, 24 December 1864, p. 720.
    (b) Notes, Queries and Replies. Med. Times and Gazette, 8 July 1865, p. 52.

11. (a) Guthrie, D.: The Renaissance of Otology. J. of Laryngology and Otology 1937; 52: 163.
    (b) Lyons, J.B.: Sir William Wilde, 1815–1876. J. Irish College of Phys. and Surgeons 1976; 5: 147.

12. The Beauties of the Boyne, Dublin: 1849.

13. Lough Corrib; Its Shores and Islands. New York: Arno Press, 1971 (reprint of 1867).

14. Irish Popular Superstitions. Totowa NJ: Rowman and Littlefield, 1973 (reprint of 1852).

Address for correspondence: Frederick C. Blodi, MD, Department of Ophthalmology, University Hospitals, Iowa City, IA 52242, USA

Documenta Ophthalmologica **81**: 75–77, 1992.
© 1992 *Kluwer Academic Publishers*.

Obituary

Noëlle Chomé-Bercioux (1898–1990), Jules Gonin's public relations' officer

JEAN F. CUENDET
Lausanne, Switzerland

A prominent lady ophthalmologist passed away. Well known by most of us, Noëlle Chomé-Bercioux, was an historical personality in the field of ophthalmology. She was Marc Dufour's Prize Laureate, Correspondent Member of the Société d'Ophtalmologie de Paris, to name but a few of her distinctions.

Long before the difficult negotiations for a European Union, Noëlle Chomé-Bercioux was already a symbol of Europe's unity. Her father was a Norman, that is French, her mother was from Lorraine, which was German until 1918 and French afterwards. By marriage she received the Luxemburg citizenship. Her step-father was Italian. Most of her studies took place

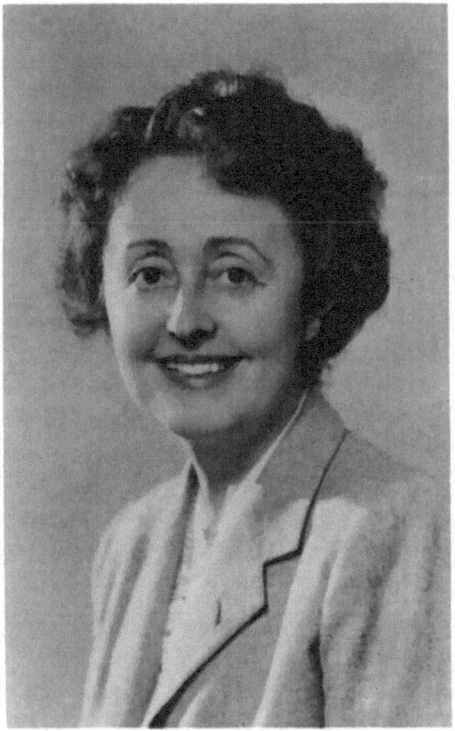

Fig. 1. Noëlle Chomé-Bercioux in 1928.

either in Austria or in Switzerland. She earned a Bachelor of Arts Degree in a convent in Fribourg, Switzerland, and then she studied engineering and mathematics at the University. Only later did she study medicine.

In 1928, Noëlle Bercioux had the great fortune to be admitted as a Resident Doctor in Professor Jules Gonin's hospital, at the very moment of the famous discovery of the surgical treatment of retinal detachment (Fig. 1).

Only a few days after her arrival in the so-called 'Asile des Aveugles' (Home for the Blind), according to Noëlle, she was introduced to three celebrities of ophthalmology: Professor Hertel from Leipzig, Germany, Professor Weill from Strassburg, France, and Docteur Ermenegildo Arruga from Barcelona, Spain. All three together with Gonin attended a surgery session with the huge thermocauter. Afterwards Gonin was too busy to take care of his hosts. So, he asked Noëlle to invite those egregious colleagues for lunch and to take them on a cruise on the Lake of Geneva to the famous castle of Chillon.

Since the discovery, more and more prominent ophthalmologists went to Lausanne (Fig. 2). Overflowed by a universal fame, Gonin committed progressively to Noëlle the care of his public relations. She owned a beautiful motorcar, something exceptional in those times. A real Lady,

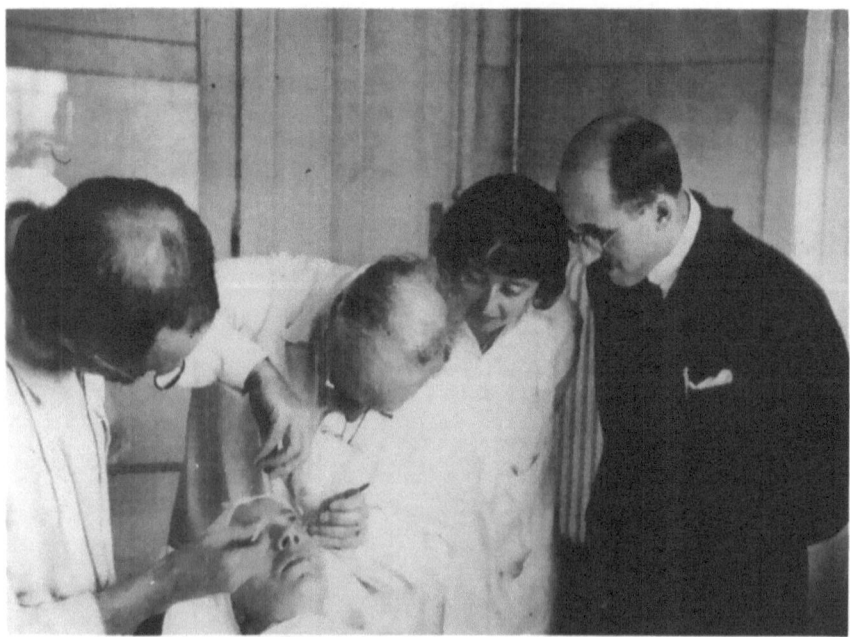

Fig. 2. Hôpital ophtalmique, Lausanne 1929: Dr. O. Dufour, Prof. J. Gonin, Dr. Noëlle Chomé-Bercioux, and Dr. Viaud.

educated at the court of her step-father the Marquis Doria,* Mrs Chomé-Bercioux excelled in this job.

The 13th International Ophthalmological Congress took place in Amsterdam, in July 1929. It enhanced the universal fame of Gonin. But although a genius, Gonin was often tired. Then, the young resident Noëlle was asked to replace him and explain his famous operation. She managed this with full success. The fame of the master shone on her. She continued to assume with efficiency Gonin's public relations' work until his death in 1936.

Furthermore, writer and journalist, Noëlle Chomé-Bercioux was a founding member of the Association suisse des Écrivains médecins (Swiss Association of Medical Writers), and later on of the World Union of Medical Writers.

In 1965, she published a memorable narration of her journey through Asia in the Trans-Siberian railway. In 1983, she published a book, entitled *Le Fous-y-tout* [Shove it all together] with a selection of her best articles, poems and bitter philosophical thoughts on retirement. She expressed her admiration of Minou Drouet, wonder child, poet, and precocious painter. She related many international conventions. She also mentioned Sir Alexander Fleming, her close friend for a few years. Nevertheless, she expressed some criticisms of his manners; he would step on her feet when dancing, and the accidental discovery of penicillin was due only to the dirtiness of Sir Alexander's laboratory.

First lady-ophthalmologist to settle down in Lausanne, she was appreciated for her very important practice. Spontaneous, generous, capricious, fashionable, worldly-minded, Noëlle Chomé-Bercioux left us an unforgettable memory of her personality.

Address for correspondence: Dr J.F. Cuendet, 31 avenue de Rumine, CH-1005 Lausanne, Switzerland.

---

*The Gotha's Calender shows that Noëlle Chomé-Bercioux's step-father Don Ernesto, Marquis Doria accumulated titles of the nobility. He was the Twelfth Principe of di Angri, the Fourth Principe di Centola, the Fifth Duca du Eboli, the Fourth Marchese de Bisciotta, the Eighth Conte du Capaccio, etc.

Documenta Ophthalmologica **81**: 79–85, 1992.

Professor Gama Pinto and
the beginning of Portuguese ophthalmology

JOÃO RIBEIRO DA SILVA

Ophthalmological Institute, Lisbon, Portugal

Gama Pinto (Fig. 1) was born in 1853 in Goa, India. He studied medicine at the Royal Medical School in Lisbon. Following his medical studies, he went to Germany where he was trained in ophthalmology under Otto Becker at the university of Heidelberg. He became 'Privat-Docent' in Heidelberg and later even Professor of Ophthalmology. In spite of this academic success, Gama Pinto always had in mind to return to his country in order to develop ophthalmology on a scientific base. Gama Pinto returned to Lisbon in 1885,

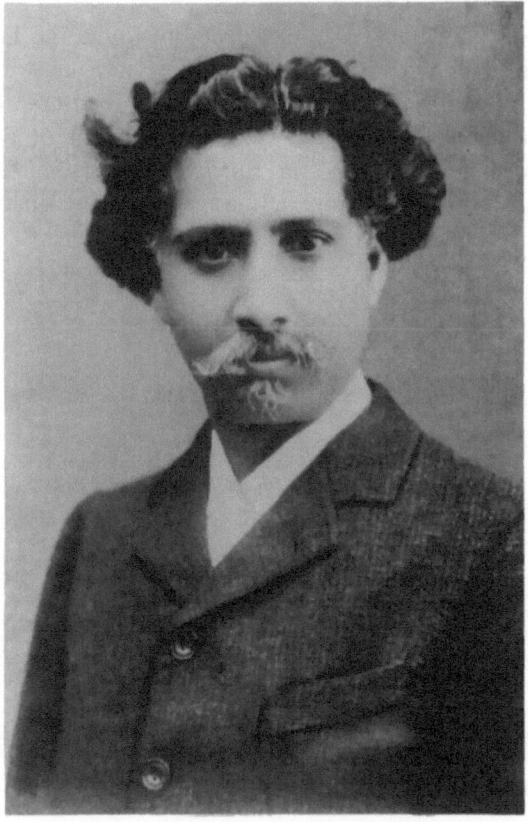

Fig. 1. Gama Pinto (1853–1945).

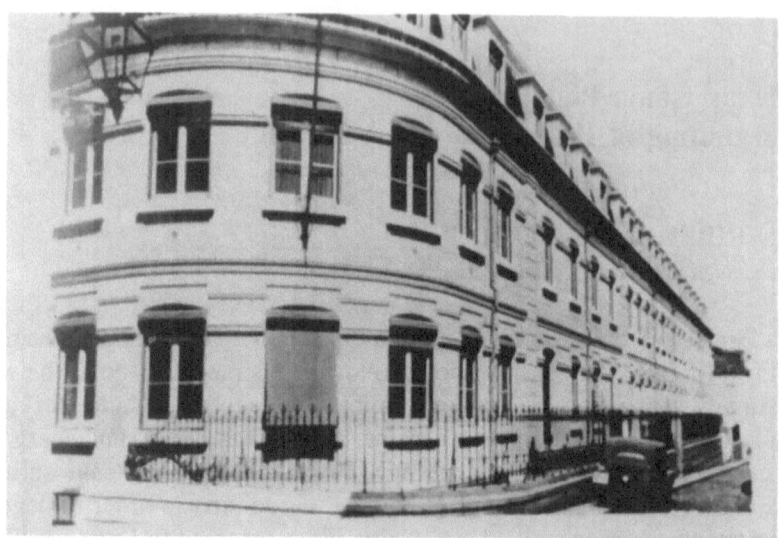

Fig. 2. The Lisbon Institute of Ophthalmology.

under the reign of King Luiz I. He proceeded to found the Lisbon Institute of Ophthalmology (Fig. 2).

In 1988 the centenary of the founding of the Institute was celebrated under the Presidency of Dr. Mario Soares, President of the Portuguese Republic (Fig. 3). The Council of the European Society of Ophthalmology was invited to attend the festivities. Among the Council members present

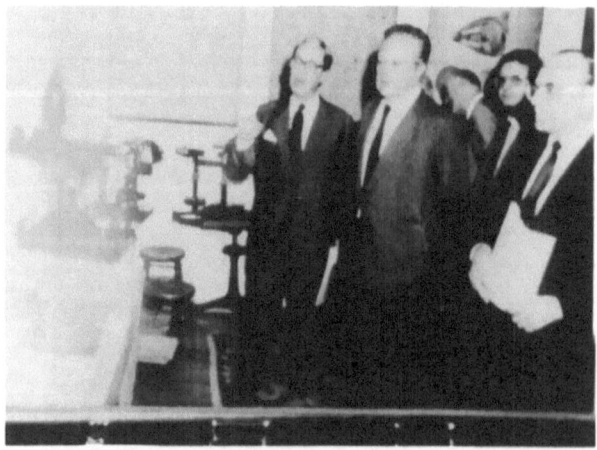

Fig. 3. The President of Portugal, Mário Soares, in the Gama Pinto Museum.

were several members of the International Academy: Saraux, Henkes, Scuderi, Meyer-Schwickerath and Theodossiadis. On that occasion, the Institute of Ophthalmology was decorated by the President of the Portuguese Republic, honouring its century of labour and scientific research.

At that time the Lisbon Institute of Ophthalmology was the only Eye Hospital and the only School of Ophthalmology in the whole country. Before Gama Pinto, there were several doctors practising ophthalmology in Lisbon and Oporto; they used to deal with eye pathology as part of general medicine and surgery. At the beginning of the 16th century, patients suffering from cataract were operated in the old hospital of 'Todos os Santos'. Famous in Europe from the 16th to the 17th centuries, this hospital was ruined in 1775 during the big earthquake that partly destroyed Lisbon.

At the beginning of the 19th century, ophthalmology was part of general medicine, at the Royal School of Medicine in Lisbon. Although, Placido da Costa deserves to be mentioned; as Professor of Physiology and of Gynecology at the Royal Medical School of Oporto, he studied ocular refraction. He developed an instrument known as 'Placido's disk', that he used for studying corneal astigmatism (Fig. 4). We still use Placido's disk as *ex libris* of the Portuguese Ophthalmological Society.

Gama Pinto, after his return from Heidelberg, became first Professor of Ophthalmology, first Director of the Lisbon Institute of Ophthalmology and, certainly, the first ophthalmological specialist of our country. In our historical and technological museum we still have the desk where Gama Pinto wrote part of his scientific papers (Fig. 5). Seated at this desk he received his patients and students. In the museum we keep several manuscripts related to his daily work in the Institute. On the wall over his desk we may see the names of those who attended the first post-graduate courses, not only in ophthalmology, but in all other medical fields, organized by Gama Pinto in 1891 (Fig. 6).

Gama Pinto brought to Portugal not only the scientific approach to ophthalmology, but also modern ideas and new methods of teaching and developing medical science.

Some of the students of the first post-graduate course became famous Portuguese doctors: Anibal Bettencourt, who was the second Director of the Bacteriological Institute of Lisbon, and Salazar de Sousa, the first professor of Pediatrics, who introduced this specialty to Portugal.

The Institute's library houses not only the papers and the books that Gama Pinto wrote, but also scientific literature from 19th century Germany, England and France (Fig. 7).

Still today it is worthwhile to read Gama Pinto's book on ocular tumors (published in 1886), as it contains very interesting histological details about retinal tumors. Gama Pinto discusses the histological characteristics of ocular tumors, their genetic and hereditary transmission, as well as their prognosis and surgical treatment.

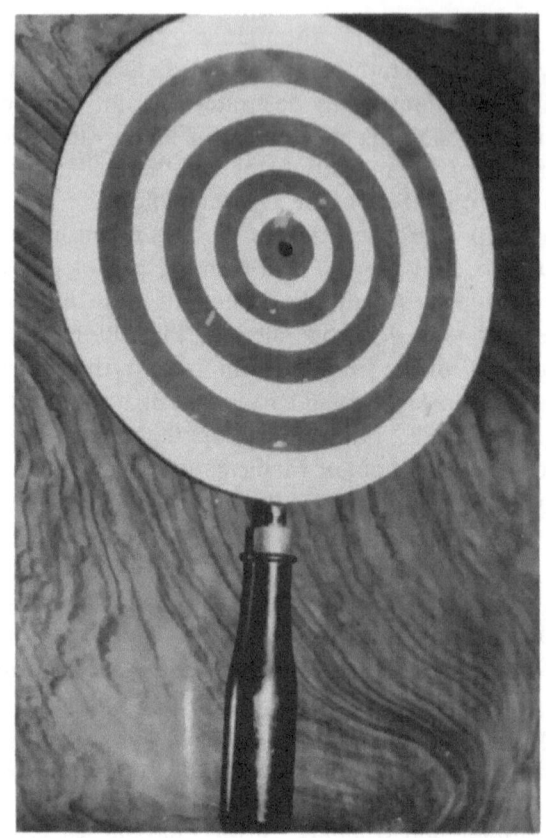

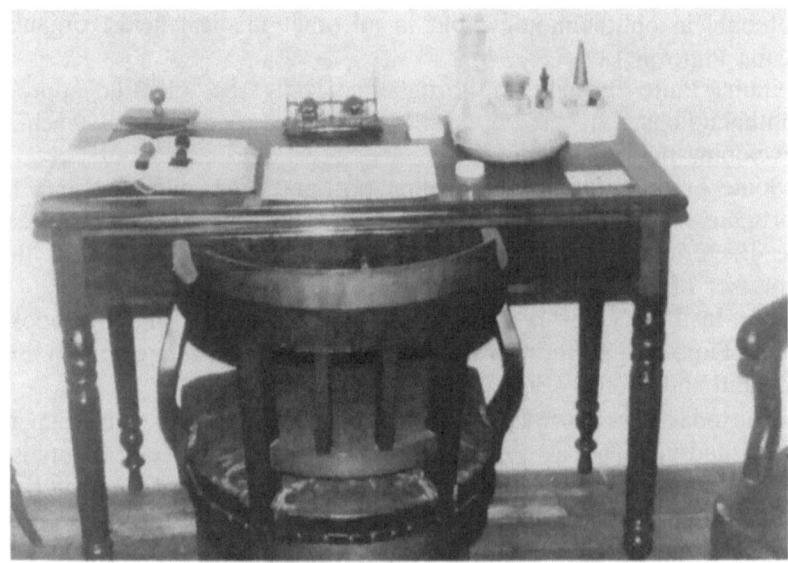

Fig. 5. The desk of Gama Pinto.

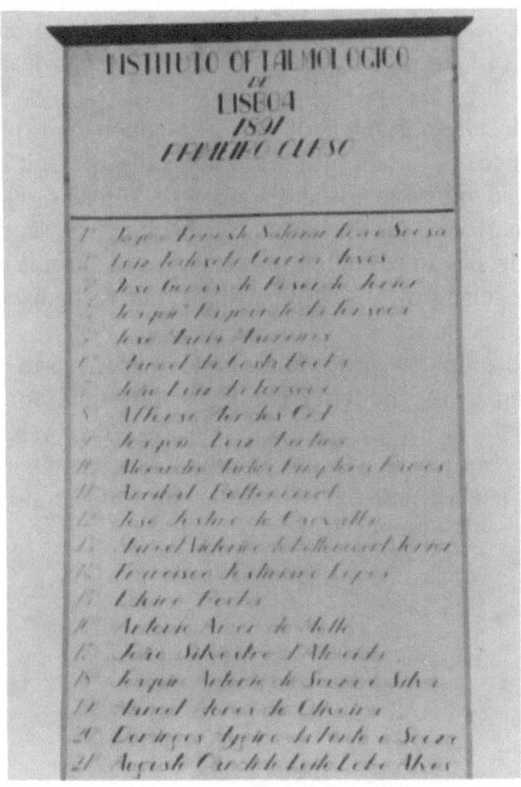

Fig. 6. The participants in the first post-graduate course in 1891.

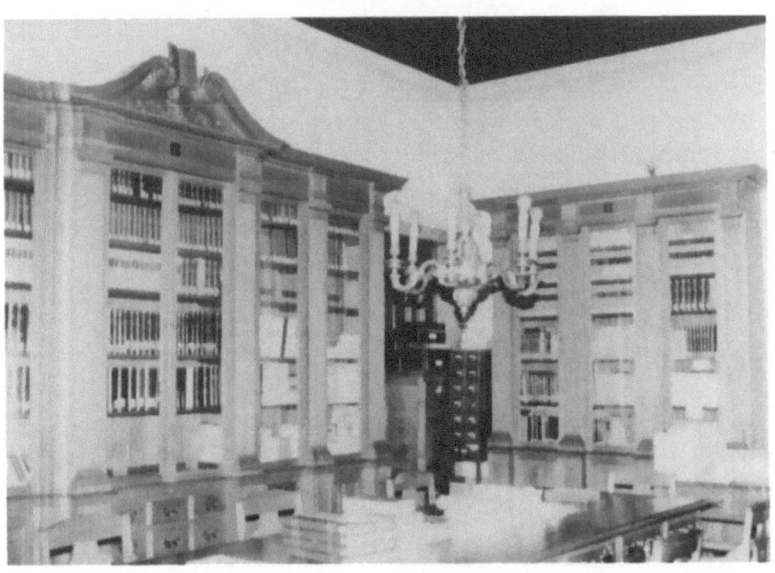

Fig. 7. The library of the Institute.

In 1900 Gama Pinto wrote a book on sympathetic ophthalmia for the French Encyclopaedia of Ophthalmology. He discussed the immunological aspects of sympathetic ophthalmia, ideas that were very advanced for that time.

Gama Pinto's most important book, in my opinion, is a book on glaucoma, also published in the French Encyclopaedia of Ophthalmology in 1900. There, Gama Pinto discussed the role of vascular sclerosis in the pathogenesis of glaucoma. According to Gama Pinto, vascular pathology can explain optic atrophy in patients with symptoms of chronic glaucoma but without high intraocular pressure. Gama Pinto thus recognized the clinical entity of low pressure glaucoma.

From the clinical point of view, Gama Pinto was an up-to-date scientist who used in his practice the modern technology of his time; for instance, for the measurement of corneal astigmatism, Placido's disk was replaced already in the 19th century by Javal's ophthalmometer. One of the first astigmometers to be constructed is kept in the Institute's museum (Fig. 8).

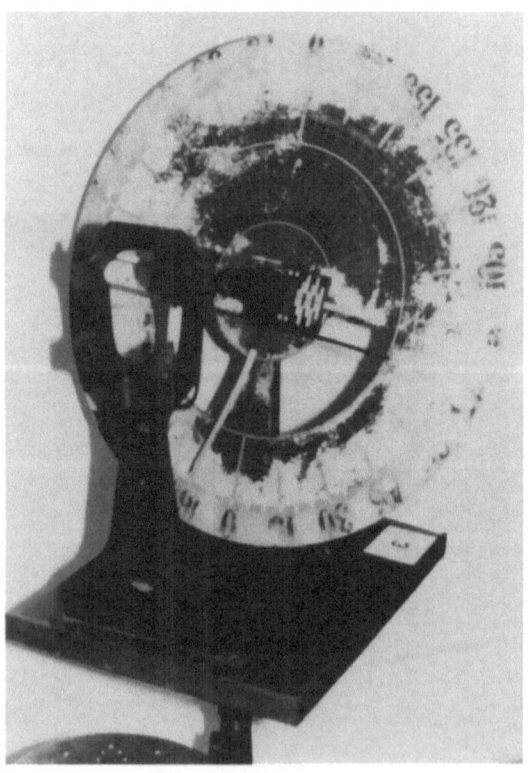

Fig. 8. An early model of Javal's ophthalmometer.

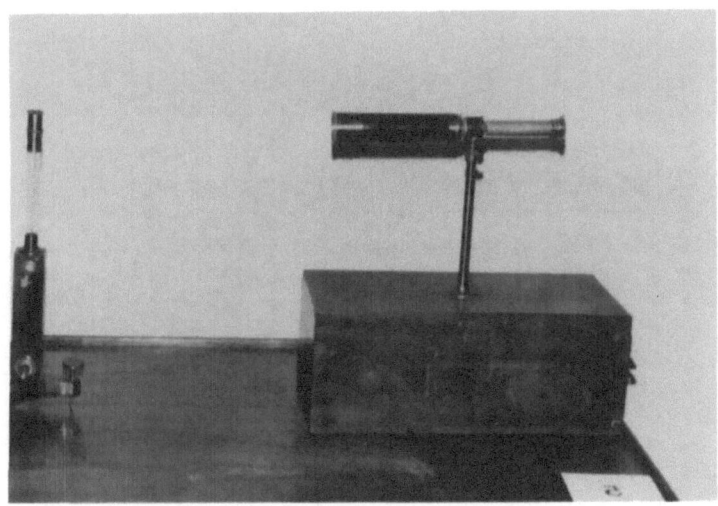

Fig. 9. Asmus's sideroscope.

Professor Gama Pinto also used the sideroscope of Asmus to diagnose intraocular magnetic foreign bodies (Fig. 9).

Gama Pinto, who died in 1945 at the age of 93, is still alive in his own Institute. He devoted his entire life to teaching ophthalmology and working on ophthalmological research. One hundred years after the founding of the Lisbon Institute of Ophthalmology, Gama Pinto's Institute continues his work.

Address for correspondence: Prof. João Ribeiro da Silva, Instituto de Oftalmologia Dr Gama Pinto, Travessa Larga 2, P-1100 Lisbon, Portugal.

Documenta Ophthalmologica **81**: 87–96, 1992.
© 1992 *Kluwer Academic Publishers*.

The first Danish Chairs of Ophthalmology

VIGGO DREYER, JENS EDMUND & P.M. MØLLER
Formerly Rigshospitalet and Copenhagen County Hospital, Copenhagen, Denmark

Key words: History of ophthalmology, Denmark, E. Hansen Grut, J. Bjerrum, M. Tscherning

Abstract. In the last century German medical sciences made up the chief inspiration to the medical profession in Europe. The influence of German ophthalmology spread to Denmark, and accordingly the first Danish professor, Edmund Hansen Grut was trained in the Graefe clinic. His successor, Jannik Bjerrum grew up in southern Jutland, a district later on lost to the German Empire. The hitherto prevailing Danish sympathies with the neighbour in the south vanished after this. Bjerrum thus wrote all his papers in Danish and made no efforts to achieve an international reputation. In contrast, Marius Tscherning, received widespread recognition as a scientist. He spent many years in France. His scientific insights at last brought him to the Danish chair of ophthalmology. The history of the first three professors of ophthalmology, so different in their attitudes, has narrative value, but exemplifies as well the rapid development of the profession in the years 1886–1925.

The year 1850 was a remarkable one in the history of ophthalmology. The first of November Albrecht von Graefe opened his out-patient clinic in a modest apartment in Berlin. December 6th Hermann von Helmholtz read his paper on his new device, the ophthalmoscope, for the Physical Society of Berlin. Two years earlier Franciscus Donders had been appointed professor 'à la suite' at the University of Utrecht, the Netherlands.*

Graefe's father, a professor of general surgery, was a skilled cataract surgeon. Twelve years old young Albrecht saw his father die, and his father's chosen profession no doubt inspired his future destiny. The genius of von Graefe, however, was his grasp of the contemporary trends which in one instant had changed ophthalmology from a purely surgical discipline to a field which encompassed the physiology and pathology of the organ of vision in total.

The fifth decade of the last century, moreover, saw the birth of European medical conferences. Physicians from several countries met to discuss their particular concerns. An ophthalmological congress in Brussels 1857 had selected Nathan Melchior, a Dane, as vice president. Melchior later became the head of the Danish Institute for the Blind, a rather provident institution. Melchior came to be an inspiration to Danish ophthalmology, and further-

---

*The term 'à la suite' implied that officially no academic position was vacant. Donders lectured on hygiene, anthropology and biology. Of outstanding interest were the courses he delivered in ophthalmology with special emphasis laid on the physiology of vision. Not before 1862 was Donders appointed to the chair of physiology of Utrecht University.

more, a personal friend of v. Graefe who married the daughter of a Danish count, Lady Anna Knuth.

Edmund Hansen Grut (1831–1907)

Edmund Gottfred Hansen was born on January 15th, 1831 in a borough of Copenhagen. In 1882 he changed his name to Hansen Grut by adding the name of his English born mother. His father was a prosperous merchant and titulary Counselor of State. In 1854 Hansen Grut graduated from the University of Copenhagen, the only one in Denmark. Three years later he defended his doctoral thesis entitled 'A short introduction to the practical use of the ophthalmoscope and some findings'. This study was based only on examination of eight patients. Its significance was more in documenting the existence of the instrument by providing original observations.

In the ensuing years Hansen Grut studied surgery and ophthalmology in

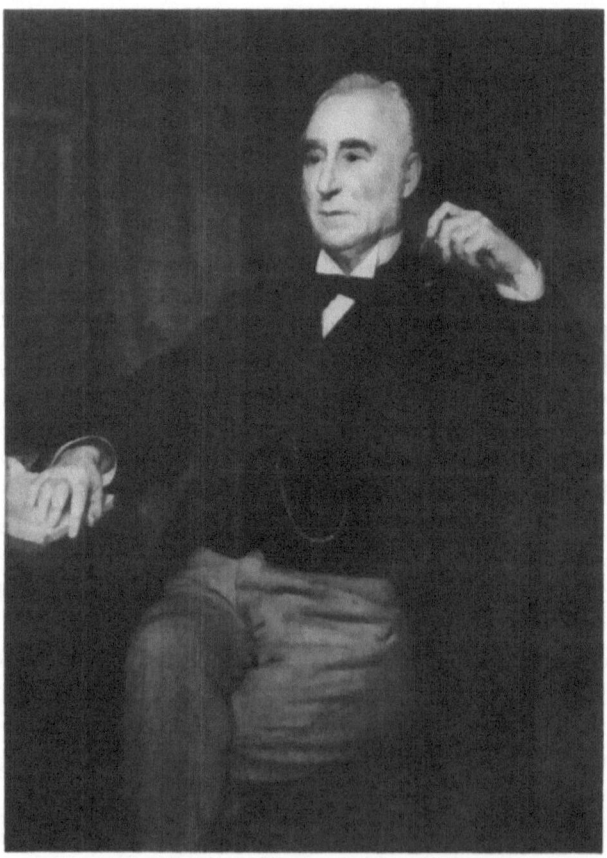

Fig. 1. Edmund Hansen Grut, 1831–1907.

Paris, London and Edinburgh. He took advice from Nathan Melchior and dedicated the year 1862 to a sojourn to Graefe's private clinic in Berlin. Although von Graefe that year had been appointed extraordinary professor of ophthalmology, seven years were to elapse, before he got his own department at the 'Charité' in Berlin.

Encouraged by ideas from the Graefe Institute, Hansen Grut the next year established his own eye clinic in Copenhagen. It was managed chiefly as an out-patient service well equipped with surgical facilities, and, in addition, with a minor ward. In the Graefe manner, the clinic offered examination and treatment free of charge to indigent people. Ten years later the clinic was better situated near the water-front of Copenhagen. This 'Harbour Street Clinic', named according to its address, subsequently became an institution well-respected in the Danish medical community everywhere outside the governing body of the university.

Here the obstinate Mathias Saxtorph, professor of general surgery held considerable power. He became the major obstacle to the adoption of ophthalmology in the university curriculum. His aversion was not due to lack of scientific activity among the clinical staff. Hansen Grut published several papers. His theoretical studies on refractive errors and accommodation were mainly surveys of Donders' research. His clinical studies were of greater value, particularly those on dendritic ulcers and bullous keratopathy.

Danish doctoral theses in those days, as still today, were defended in public before two critics or referees, appointed by the dean of the medical school. At such an academic session a young doctor presented his treatise on glaucoma. Professor Saxtorph, official critic, here expressed this dictum: 'The new development within ophthalmology must be denoted as charlatism!' This declaration prompted Hansen Grut to reply, and he wrote a contribution entitled 'Objection' in the principal Danish medical journal. Here he pointed out that a university professor, still reasonably young, must be required to possess qualifications to control his own petrification. Furthermore, the adoption of exclusive and strongly individual attitudes presumes a unique scientific capacity, hitherto not demonstrated by Professor Saxtorph. These harsh remarks did not benefit the introduction of the new medical discipline.

The Faculty of Medicine on the other hand supported Hansen Grut and acknowledged his scientific capability. In the following years a lengthy discussion began between the faculty and university authorities. As a member of the faculty, P.L. Panum, the well known physiologist, in 1870 proposed the establishment of a ward for the eye diseases in the Royal Frederik's Hospital, the Danish University Hospital. Panum, too, met resistance. Eventually, the faculty suggested the establishment of a training program in ophthalmology outside the university's campus. The service was to remain in Harbour Street, now well staffed and equipped. Aside from patient fees, Hansen Grut would be offered a compensation for expenses connected with the running of the clinic. Again the university refused. The administration wrote that no convincing reasons could be found to divide medicine into tiny parts which would result in the loss of a comprehensive medical outlook. The next step would be university chairs for masseurs and chiropodists.

The dean of the medical school replied in drastic terms that despite its minor volume, the exact knowledge of the function of the eyeball was paramount in medicine.

At last common sense gained victory. In the years 1871 to 1882 Hansen Grut gave private lectures, and in 1882 he was appointed temporary lecturer at the university. Six years later he took office as the first Danish professor of ophthalmology, and an arrangement was adopted which transferred the training of undergraduates to his private clinic. During his tenure he asserted his authority firmly and discouraged opposition against his clinical or administrative ideas. He retired in the year 1896 and became honorary member of the Danish Ophthalmological Society, founded in the year 1900. Hansen Grut died in 1907.

Jannik Bjerrum (1851–1920)

Jannik Petersen Bjerrum became the second Danish professor of Ophthalmology. While the obstacles to the appointment of the first professor mainly were focused upon the actual need for the establishment of the chair, the issue now focused on the selection of one of three applications. The ultimate choice, however, had to be made between Tscherning and Bjerrum. Marius Tscherning for many years had lived in Paris, and his research had established his international reputation. His ability as a clinician on the other hand was less outstanding. Bjerrum, in contrast, had worked all his professional life in the Harbour Street Clinic under the guidance of Hansen Grut, who sincerely wished to select his successor. At that time Bjerrum was the senior assistant and joint owner of the clinic. During the appointment procedures Hansen Grut issued a declaration that if Bjerrum did not obtain the ophthalmological chair, the Harbour Street Clinic would no longer serve as a university clinic. Indeed this was a very strong argument in favour of Bjerrum, and under these circumstances no one could be surprised that Bjerrum was appointed the chair.

Anyhow, these unfortunate events were regrettable and unnecessary since Bjerrum was an excellent ophthalmologist and a serious scientist who probably would have done well without these maneuvers.

Jannik Petersen Bjerrum was born December 26th 1851 in Skarbak, a village in the most southern part of Jutland in the border district between the Danish kingdom and the Duchy of Schleswig-Holstein. This was a highly disputed area and the object of numerous political debates and military battles. In 1848 just before Bjerrum was born, a local rebellion evolved into a war between the Danish king and the German-oriented duke. This war

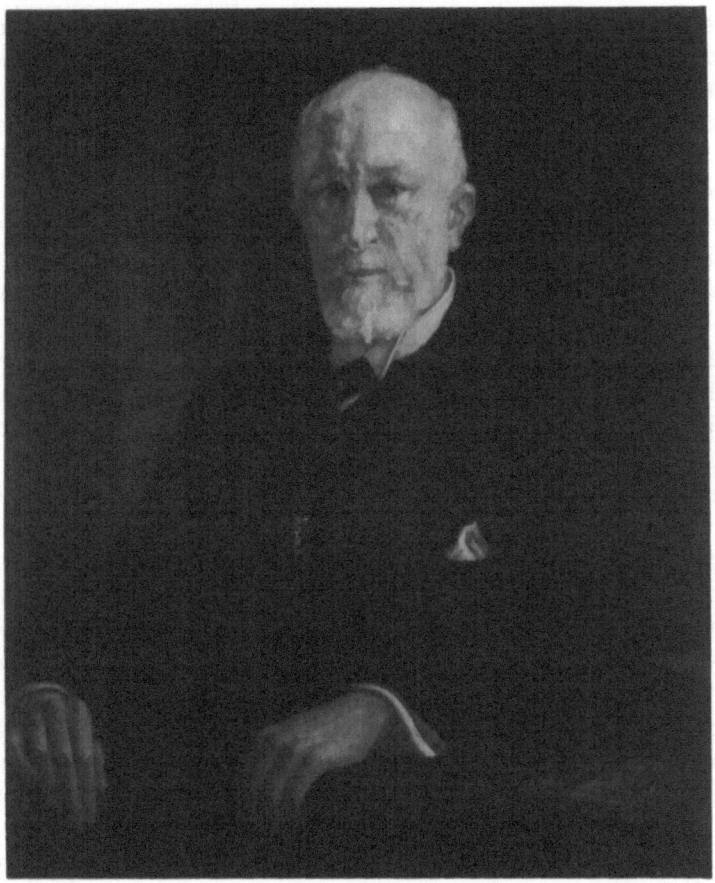

Fig. 2. Jannik Bjerrum, 1851–1920.

ended with a glorious Danish victory, and Schleswig-Holstein remained a part of Denmark, but only for a short period. In 1864 another war started, now between Germany (and Austria) and Denmark. In short order this campaign ended in a total Danish defeat, and southern Jutland, almost one third of the kingdom, was incorporated in the new German Empire where it remained until 1920. Thus Bjerrum was born in Denmark, but grew up in Germany.

He left the Cathedral School of Ribe, Denmark in 1869 and completed his medical degree in 1876 in Copenhagen. Inspired by Hansen Grut he soon became interested in ophthalmology and was appointed Hansen Grut's assistant in 1879. Bjerrum's scientific concern was the relationship between visual perception of form and the resolving power in localized areas of the retina. He demonstrated this in his thesis entitled 'Undersøgeleser over Formsans og Lyssans i forskellige Øjensygdomme' (Investigations on the form sense and light sense in various eye diseases). This title is deliberately given in Danish to indicate that through his entire lifetime it was mandatory for Bjerrum to write his publications in Danish. An antipathy against German, in those days the language of science, may have been gained in a childhood so filled with tensions regarding nationalism.

The scientific achievement that made the name Bjerrum universally known was conceived during his work on the relationship between visual acuity and the perception of the bright stimuli in various retinal zones. In accordance with his own modest attitude, this discovery was published in 1889 in a small paper which in translation was called 'An addendum to the usual examination of the visual field of glaucoma'. At that time Bjerrum was studying the visual field by means of small white objects. The idea of this investigation was to record the performance of every single functional unit of the retina. As a minimum such units in Bjerrum's opinion would subtend a visual angle of one minute of arc (in the macular region). However, even a small test object would subtend a visual angle exceeding two degrees and accordingly cover a multitude of functional units. In order to obtain a better functional portrayal of the retina, Bjerrum conceived the idea of enlarging the observation distance. Initially, a standard perimetry was carried out by the aid of a perimeter arc with a radius of 30 cm and a 10 mm test object. A screen was placed next to the perimeter arc. The subsequent step was to move the chinrest table backwards to an observation distance of two meters and plot the visual field on the screen without the use of the perimeter arc. In this case an object of 3 mm was employed. This last procedure was the first introduction of campimetry, which eventually gained worldwide use. By campimetry Bjerrum demonstrated the very small glaucomatous scotomas later called the scotoma of Bjerrum in recognition of its discoverer.

During his tenure as professor beginning in 1896 Bjerrum directed the still private clinic on Harbour Street. Although he possessed limited ability as a teacher, he impressed his students with his clinical honesty and the integrity of his scientific work. In his personal dealings and in his clinical and scientific work he displayed an impressive logic and intelligence, but never lost his modesty. His never failing responsibility formed a fashion for the coming generation of Danish ophthalmologists.

In 1910 when aged 59 years Bjerrum retired but continued to reside in Copenhagen. As previously mentioned, his origin from Schleswig remained important to him all of his life and resulted in a substantial national feeling that made him feel it a duty and honour to publish his scientific works in Danish to avoid confusion with alien research. The scientific community fully realized that this was a Danish paper.

His national attitude also led to one of his final decisions. The termination of the first World War and the collapse of the German Empire brought to the fore the matter of the occupied southern border districts in the post-war peace conference. In 1920, a referendum was initiated to give the inhabitants of Schleswig the opportunity to choose their future homeland. The electorate was those born in the district. Already a sick and old man, Bjerrum went from Copenhagen to his native village to give his vote, and in this way he contributed to the homecoming of Schleswig to the Danish kingdom. Jannik Petersen Bjerrum died the same year.

Marius Tscherning (1854–1939)

Hans Erik Marius Tscherning was born December 11, 1854 as a son of a school teacher in a small village near Odense, also known as the native town of Hans Christian Andersen. He graduated from medical school in Copenhagen in 1878, and four years later he defended his doctoral thesis titled 'On the etiology of myopia'. This study was rather outstanding by contemporary standards. During service for the draft board, Tscherning evaluated the fitness of 7564 conscripts and took the opportunity to ascertain their refractive errors. This procedure was conducted by the aid of an ophthalmoscope, and, second to none, he maintained the skill to do so throughout all his lifetime. Hansen Grut had encouraged him to initiate the

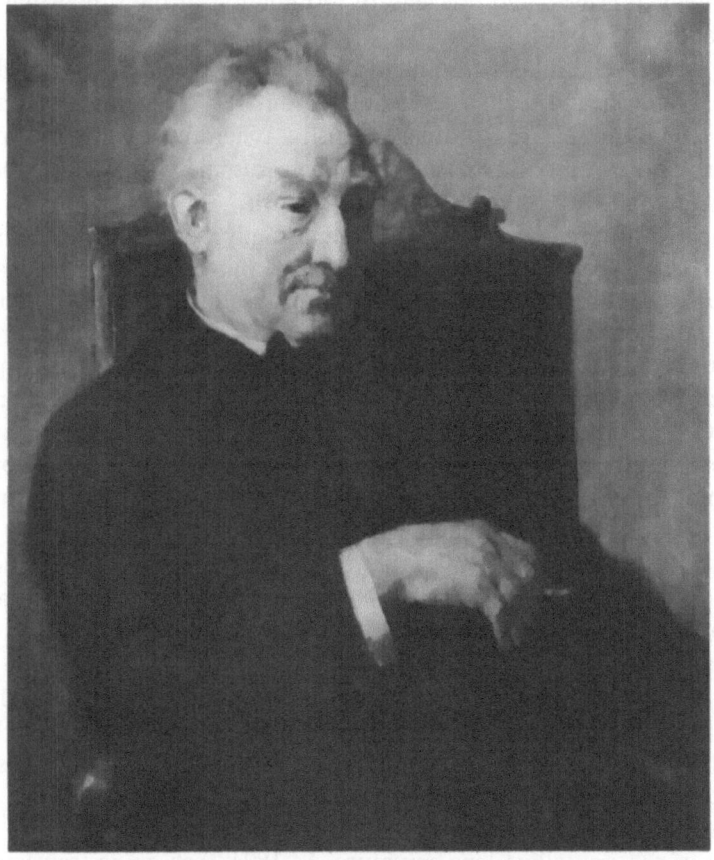

Fig. 3. Marius Tscherning, 1854–1939.

investigation and furthermore offered him employment as an assistant in his clinic. However, a disagreement arose between the scholar and his tutor as to conclusions to be drawn from the study. Hansen Grut held the common opinion that myopia resulted from reading. Tscherning, on the other hand, felt that the issue was more complicated. As a matter of fact he demonstrated that the prevalence of myopia was not equally stratified in various social groups. In credit to the school myopia theory, however, he found myopia to be most common among high school students.

Tscherning undertook brief study tours to Berlin and Cologne, and ultimately to Paris. In 1884 he succeeded in obtaining a post as deputy director at the Visual Research Institute of the University of Sorbonne. In this position he followed Hjalmar Schiøtz, the Norwegian who became the father of the tonometer. Tscherning spent the next 26 years in Paris. The senior director, Emile Javal had qualified for degrees in technology as well as in medicine. He inspired his students to serious scientific achievements, but eventually he changed his concern from visual sciences to political affairs, as he became a member of the French Chamber of Deputies. This engagement, however, did not lead to termination of the supporting grants to his laboratory, but had the opposite effect.

Javal gave Tscherning a free hand to carry out research and taught him academic French and Gallic perfection. Ultimately Tscherning was said to have become more French than Danish. When he finally returned to Denmark and assumed his position as professor, he wrote his textbook in French, thereafter to be translated into Danish.

Emil Javal suffered from glaucoma and virtually went blind before he died in 1901. That year Tscherning assumed the full control of the institute. Unfortunately, this promotion did not improve his standards of living. In fact he experienced an unjustly meager existence during his voluntary exile in Paris and had to supplement his poor income with earnings from private practice. While still in charge Javal often discussed the establishment of a chair at the Sorbonne for his deputy director. These great expectations, however, never were fulfilled. Nor was this his first dashed hope, as Tscherning experienced earlier disappointment in 1896 when Bjerrum was appointed the chair of ophthalmology in Copenhagen.

Science remained the driving force of his life. His research was devoted almost exclusively to visual science. He collected his Sorbonne lectures in a textbook entitled 'Optique physiologique' which obtained widespread recognition.

Prior to his stay in Paris he had already shown interest in the mechanism of accommodation, encouraged by the works of Thomas Young, the British ophthalmologist and gifted mathematician. Although known for his color vision theory, Young in 1801 published a paper 'On the mechanism of the eye', as well. Here he described the nature of accommodation to be an increase of the crystalline lens curvature. In 1894 Tscherning translated and commented on Young's treatise.

In a paper from 1895 he contrasted the theories of Donders and Helm-holtz. The study was experimental and the features of accommodation were ascertained from the Pukinje images reflected from the front and back surfaces of the crystalline lens. In his autobiography Tscherning mentions that his wife served as an excellent subject in these sittings as she taught herself to accommodate on command. His accommodation theories, how-ever, did not meet general acceptance, and even his countrymen felt that only a fool could oppose Helmholtz's dogmatism.

Another research objective was the study of the optics of spectacle lenses. Trials had already rendered it reasonable that meniscus glasses that re-spected the gaze rotations of the eyeball should be preferred to bi-convex glasses. Tscherning laid down an equation of second degree, the two solutions of which were in accordance with the two sets of results hitherto obtained empirically. Tscherning handed over his formulas to a French manufacturer. Concurrently, Alvar Gullstrand, the Swedish ophthalmologist and Nobel laureate, applied to the Carl Zeiss Works in Jena with his version. He attended Tscherning's presentation of his paper and his contri-bution was an improvement of the formulas to cover a larger range of powers. So it happened that Gullstrand's name was attributed to the 'Puntalgalser' and 'Cathralglaser' marketed by Zeiss. Eventually Tscherning was acknowledged as the originator, but Gullstrand and Tscherning never became friends.

1910 came to be the year when circumstances formally favored Tscher-ning's scientific endeavors. That year a new University Hospital (Rigshos-pitalet) was built, and Bjerrum was reluctant to change his position. Tscherning applied for the chair and was appointed without the academic competition so common in those days.

He was soon recognized as an inspiring teacher. He trained his students in front of the 'optical bench' located in the basement of the eye department. This served as his workshop and was well equipped with instruments brought home from Paris and still in use many years after his retirement in 1925. Here he gave inspiration to the new generation of ophthalmologists and initiated new research fields, particularly on the adaptation of retina. These experiments were conducted by virtue of his logarithmic filters, the photometric glasses.

Tscherning, kind and with a common touch, was popular with staff and patients. His vivid appearance, his great white mane, and his artist's bow ties can be recalled by two of the authors of this paper (JE and PMM). As children they dropped in and enjoyed sweets from his desk drawer. Marius Tscherning died in 1939.

The incumbents of the first three chairs had very dissimilar attitudes. Hansen Grut was the polemic executive of an eye clinic of his own making. Bjerrum made enduring discoveries but was never anxious for fame. Marius Tscherning believed substantially in science, but his enthusiasm, had to

96

sustain him through some major disappointments. All three saw a rapid development in ophthalmology and observed theories rise and decline. In his memoirs Tscherning concluded that the very truth is the ever changing truth.

References

Bjerrum J: Bemærkninger om Formindskelsen af Synsstyrken. Nord. ophth. Tidskr. 1889; I(2): 95.

Bjerrum J: Om en Tilføjelse til den sædvanlige Synsfeltsundersøgelse. Nord. ophth. Tidskr. 1889; II(3): 141.

Hansen E: Indsigelse. Hospitalstid. 1867; 10: 29.

Hansen E: Om Refraktions- og Akkommodationsanomalier. Bibl. f. Læger 1863; VI(5): 1.

Kugelberg F: Albrecht von Graefe och hans tid. Stockholm: Gebers, 1950.

Lottrup-Andersen Chr: Det ophthalmologiske selskab i Københavns historie Bibl. f. Læger; 1952: aug.

Norrie G: Den Danske Oftalmologis Historie. Copenhagen: Levin & Munksgaard, 1925.

Rønne H: Über Ordination anastigmatischer und orthoskopischer Brillengläser. Klin. Monatsbl. 1917; 58: 285.

Tscherning M: Studier over Myopiens Ætiologi. Copenhagen: C. Myhre, 1882.

Tscherning M: Le mécanisme de l'accommodation. Ann. d'ocul. 1904; 131: 1.

Tscherning M: Optique physiologique Paris: Carré et Naud, 1898.

Ugeskr. f. Læger (Editorial) 1881; 4(3): 1.

Address for correspondence: Prof. Dr Viggo Dreyer, Frederiksgade 10, DK-1265 Copenhagen K, Denmark.

Documenta Ophthalmologica **81**: 97–101, 1992.

Ophthalmology in Europe
in the days of the French Revolution

P. BREGEAT(†) & P. AMALRIC
Centre Médical Ophtalmologique, Albi, France

Key words: History of ophthalmology, optics, French Revolution, 18th century

Abstract. The authors highlight the political and scientific landmarks in 18th century France; the Revolution of 1789 had positive effects, in that it marked the accession of the French middle-class to political power and enabled the promotion of young scientists without consideration of social class or fortune; it had negative effects, in that France lost the scientific edge it had gained when all existing chairs in ophthalmology were abolished. The status of ophthalmology and of physiological optics in the 18th century are discussed, with a brief mention of the most important innovators in the field.

The celebration of the Bicentennial of the French Revolution was the occasion for important cultural events in France and in numerous other countries. The history of this period has often been related, as the French Revolution greatly influenced many fields, among which science and culture. However, having consulted numerous books and papers on this subject [1–4, 7–11], we may really wonder to what extent the French Revolution was actually worth-while.

On 14 July 1989, magnificent celebrations have marked the anniversary of the Declaration of Human Rights. Nevertheless, it has been pointed out that this major event had been preceded not only by the Magna Carta in England, but also by the Declaration of Independence of United States.

The first stages of the French Revolution correspond to a transformation of mentalities and above all marked the accession of the French middle-class to political power. The fall of the Bastille and the first years of Revolution were saluted with enthusiasm in Europe.

The Age of Enlightenment, represented by great encyclopedists as Voltaire, Diderot, d'Alembert and Buffon had prepared this change but the total destruction of a political system had not been planned. After Louis XVI had finally admitted these reforms, most people thought that everything was settled and that France could start off again to a still more brilliant future. French language was commonly used at the courts of Frederick II of Prussia, Maria-Theresia of Austria and Catherine II of Russia. Frontiers did not exist and, if we want to summarize the situation in one sentence, we could say that, in the 18th century, Paris had become the capital of Europe.

The American writer Charles Coulston Gillispie [5], who undertook a large study on sciences in France at the end of the 18th century, notes that no country had such a complete structure of universities as France. The foundation of the Society of Medicine counterbalanced the too rigid dogmatism of the Faculty and prefigured the present National Academy of Medicine. Natural history was taught at the College of France and, for the most part, at the Jardin du Roi where men as Buffon, Jussieu, Daubanton or Lamarck conveyed a very substantial knowledge.

Finally, ophthalmology was recognized as a specialty, at least as concerns its clinical teaching; the victory of surgical ideas initiated by Daviel was progressively confirmed. The operation of cataract was still discussed but, little by little, the technique of extraction was practically admitted by the quasi totality of enlightened Europe.

Though physiology and optics were not integrated into ophthalmology, examination with the lens or the microscope yielded a more precise knowledge of the anatomy of the eye.

The relations between universities were frequent: the Latin language, commonly spoken and written by all, facilitated the diffusion of ideas from England to Germany and from Italy to France. We shouldn't say that everything was then perfect but great personalities emerged from the European universities of Leiden, London, Göttingen, Pavia and Bologna. In France, Louis XVI founded the first two European clinics of ophthalmology in Paris and Montpellier.

Of course, some have assumed that great political revolutions have given rise to fundamental scientific discoveries. This theory was applied to England as concerns Charles I's death which was considered as having generated Harvey's discoveries and Newton's theories on light and universal gravitation. But to establish a correlation between political events and scientific discoveries is rather hazardous and numerous examples do not confirm this hypothesis. And this is particularly true as regards the French Revolution. From a chronological point of view, it occurred at the end of a period which was particularly rich in political and cultural events, and which also bordered on a century of considerable discoveries.

The end of the 18th century had been marked by significant advances in medical knowledge. Yet, the medicine of systems was still persistent and provoked long debates of ideas in Germany with Stahl, Hahnemann and later Mesmer and his pupils, in England with Brown and Cullen, in France with Bordere and Boutler at Montpellier, Cabanes in Paris, and in Italy with Rosari and Thomasini.

The theories of systems began to be confronted with an anatomo-clinical method which was initiated by a man of genius: Giovanni Morgagni, a pupil of Malpighi and Valsalva, who is considered as one of the founders of pathological anatomy. By the end of the 18th century, Italy was at the top level of scientific progress and Scarpa, Galvani, Volta, Panizza, Rolando are among its great scientists. In Edinburgh, Halle and Monroe were very famous and, in the Netherlands, the school of Leiden was preeminent.

Progress was constant; dogmatism did not impede scientific development based on anatomical and physiological studies. Great European sovereigns as Catherine II of Russia, Frederick II of Prussia, Joseph II in Austria, Georges III in England, the popes in Italy and the French kings promoted the great academic institutions in their respective countries and honoured great scholars and scientists who contributed to important achievements.

At that time, ophthalmology did not correspond to what it is today. The study of optics and light phenomena was always the prerogative of physicians and philosophers. Experimentation was performed in laboratories of physics where the medical doctor did not in fact play the part of initiator.

The problems of optical glasses were often solved by empirical methods and only myopia and presbyopia could be so corrected. Janin wrote several publications on strong hypermetropia but no optical explanation was given; the same was the case for astigmatism.

The figure of Newton reigns over the whole century. His corpuscular theories on light were not contested. Despite the difficulties they imply to explain some phenomena, they remain the Bible of scientists. However, since Grimaldi and Huyghens' works, the undulatory theory always had its adepts. Goethe was violently opposed to Newton as regards the theory of colours. Moreover in France, Marat, the revolutionary Doctor in Edinburgh, challenged the accuracy of the seven fundamental colours and definitely recognized only three of them.

At that period, an ophthalmological examination did not include the study of refraction, though knowledge of the anatomy of the eye had significantly improved since the beginning of the century. The ophthalmometric investigations on frozen eyeballs by Pourfour du Petit constitute the first biometric study performed not only in humans but also in animals. In his work on cataract, Brisseau designed anatomical cuts which are correct as concerns the location of intraocular elements. Surgical knowledge was rather limited to the operation of the cataract and lacrimal fistula. In that field, Daviel had established a new and original technique which was followed by several schools in France and in Germany.

Ophthalmology was developing into a medical specialty which was studied by several schools: in Italy at Pavia, in Austria at Vienna, and in France at Paris and Montpellier. Itinerant ophthalmologists were still travelling all through Europe; Taylor and Pellier de Quengsy are the most famous, and numerous ophthalmological books and treatises were published.

To define this period, we should refer to Hirschberg's comments [6] according to which the 18th century was the century of Renaissance in ophthalmology and the great century of French ophthalmology. But the French Revolution led to a total transformation of society, to the dissolution of existing scientific structures and to the suppression of all chairs of medicine which, according to the revolutionary concept, were too much linked with the Ancien Régime and had to be suppressed. For this reason, all chairs of ophthalmology disappeared and France lost the edge it had gained.

In all fields, men who had been at the origin of important discoveries were not completely removed from the scientific scene and they continued to provide their knowledge to the political power. Of course, the defense of the nation against all the rest of Europe was then primordial.

By contrast with numerous officers and sailors who emigrated, scientists did not leave the country; they took part in numerous organizations – some did it with enthusiasm but others, as Lavoisier, were the victims of revolutionary passion.

Nevertheless, most members of the Academy of Sciences were nominated in the first promotion of members of the Institute of France. Just after the fall of Robespierre at Thermidor and under the Directory or the Consulate, the scientific structures were often organized on the same basis as under the royalty.

The main merit of this period was to enable the promotion of young scientists without consideration of social class or fortune. Compulsory education with the creation of colleges as well as the foundation of the Polytechnic School were going to give rise to a generation of new scientists who were to work mostly in the field of physics and optics: Malus, Biot, Arago and later Fresnel.

At that period, ophthalmology was not considered as a medical priority. Numerous generalist surgeons operated cataracts and treated ocular problems; many of them, who belonged to the Army, distinguished themselves during the Napoleonic wars; Scarpa in Pavia, Forlenze in Roma and Quadri contributed to place Italy in an eminent rank at the beginning of the 19th century.

In Mainz, Germany, Soemmering influenced Larrey through his teaching and his treatises; he collaborated on a work with Demours.

In England, a young man of genius named Thomas Young realized the most exhaustive study of the eye including its sensory physiology and physiologic optics. He asserted his opposition to Newton's theories by confirming Huygens' hypothesis of the undulatory transmission of light. Severely criticized in England, Arago and Fresnel performed experiments in Paris which confirmed Young's studies and marked the starting point of a new theory of colour vision which is still recognized.

In Western Europe, the beneficial contribution of doctors in ophthalmology stands in sharp contrast to the murderous madness of men animated by the revolutionary spirit. It is not possible to associate their discoveries with the course of political events; the primacy of individual genius in the creation of original works must be acknowledged.

Actually, the political revolution has never corresponded with the scientific revolution. Genius consists in a personal opposition to the belief of the masses and to accepted theories. Men cannot be defined in relation to the events or periods they live through. When they think counter to the usual theories, they may sometimes be confronted with dramatic situations or even become martyrs, as was the case for Galileo, Young, Einstein, Darwin, Semmelweis, to name but a few famous figures of science. Others such as Mendel or Purkinje, were unknown to their contemporaries. In most cases, official praise is long overdue. Great scientists are often in opposition to their contemporaries and to their times.

References

1. Barthelemy, Guy: Les savants sous la Révolution. Le Mans: Ed. Cénomane, 1988.
2. Besset, Florence and Beaujard, Yves: Les savants et la Révolution (Coll. Monde en Poche). Paris: Ed. Nathan, 1989.
3. Cohen, J. Bernard: Revolution in Science. Cambridge: The Belknap Press of Harvard University Press, 1985.
4. Dhombres, Nicole: Les savants en Révolution 1789–1799. Paris: Calmann-Lévy, 1989.
5. Gillispie, Charles C.: Science and Polity in France at the end of the Old Regime Princeton: Princeton University Press, 1980.
6. Hirschberg, J.: Handbuch der Gesamten Augenheilkunde. Geschichte der Augenheilkunde IX & X: Die Reform der Augenheilkunde. Berlin: J. Springer, 1918.
7. Guedj, Denis: La Révolution des savants (Coll. Découvertes). Paris: Gallimard, 1989.
8. Rashed, R.: Sciences à l'époque de la Révolution Française (Recherches historiques). Paris: A. Blanchard, 1988.
9. Sournia, Jean-Charles: La médecine révolutionnaire (1789–1799). Paris: Ed. Payot, 1989.
10. Tulard, J., Fayard, J.F., Fierro, A.: Histoire et dictionnaire de la Révolution Française 1789–1799. Paris: R. Laffont, 1987.
11. La Révolution Française et l'Europe 1789–1799. Paris: Ed. de la Réunion des Musées nationaux, 1989.

Address for correspondence: Prof. Pierre Amalric, MD, Centre Médical Ophtalmologique, 6 rue Saint-Clair, F-81000 Albi, France.

Documenta Ophthalmologica **81**: 103–109, 1992.
© 1992 *Kluwer Academic Publishers*.

The present status of the Hirschberg Library

AKIRA NAKAJIMA & SHIZU SAKAI
Juntendo University, Tokyo, Japan

Key words: History of ophthalmology, Hirschberg (1843–1925), Germany, Japan

Professor Hirschberg was born in Potsdam on 18 September 1843 and died on 17 February 1925 in Berlin. He studied ophthalmology under Albrecht von Graefe. He became 'Ausserordentlicher Professor' of ophthalmology at the University of Berlin in 1879, and honorary professor in 1890. He introduced the use of a strong electromagnet for removing magnetic foreign bodies from the eye. He founded the *Zentralblatt für Augenheilkunde* in 1877, and looked after it for 43 years [1].

What made Hirschberg world famous were his library and his contribution to the history of ophthalmology in Graefe Saemisch's *Handbuch der gesammten Augenheilkunde*, published in 9 volumes in 1899–1918. His 'opus magnum' on the history of ophthalmology in Graefe Saemisch's *Handbuch* was recently translated into English by Dr. Blodi.* Some time ago a discussion started, how to extend Hirschberg's History of Ophthalmology to include the 20th century. As the amount of publications increases exponentially with time, this will be really a tough job.

Some years ago, we published an article on the Hirschberg Library [2]. Recently, Dr. Blodi asked me about the present status of the Library. It is located in the Central Library of the University of Tokyo. I went there to see whether the Hirschberg Library was still in good condition.

Present status of the Hirschberg Library

The Central Library of the University of Tokyo was built in 1892. At that time, it was one of the best equipped university libraries with 400 000 books and 300 seats spread over 1440 square meters. The big earthquake in Tokyo on 1 September 1923 completely destroyed the building. The books burned down in the fire which broke out just after the earthquake. The whole collection of books built up over the past thirty years had become ash in a matter of hours.

---

*At present, Dr. F.C. Blodi, Department of Ophthalmology, University of Iowa, USA, is preparing a detailed bibliography on Hirschberg.

The rebuilding of the library, completed in 1928, was possible by the donation of 4 million yen (more than 40 million US dollars in present currency) by the Rockefeller Foundation. For that reason the present library is nicknamed 'Rockefeller Library' (Fig. 1). Great Britain and other countries donated 300 000 books. Donations in Japan amounted to 200 000; purchases by the budget of the library numbered 100 000, totalling 600 000 books. The numbers should have increased by now. The above information was taken from a booklet by Yoshio Ando [3] published on the occasion of the 50th anniversary of the Library after the restoration.

The Hirschberg Library became famous through the publication of a catalogue in 1901. In its preface, Hirschberg stated that the library was to be donated to the Berlin Medical Society. The catalogue had a subject index as well as an author index.

Hirschberg travelled around the world in 1892 and wrote a book *Reise um die Erde* about his travels. He stayed in Japan in September 1892. He visited various places in Japan, and had a good time with Dr. Scriba, who taught ophthalmology at the University of Tokyo at that time. He met many other Japanese ophthalmologists. He may have received a nice impression about Japan.

In 1921 he wrote a letter to Prof. Komoto, at that time the Head of the Department of Ophthalmology at Tokyo University, offering his library for 40 000 yen, in present currency 400 000 US dollars. Prof. Komoto decided to

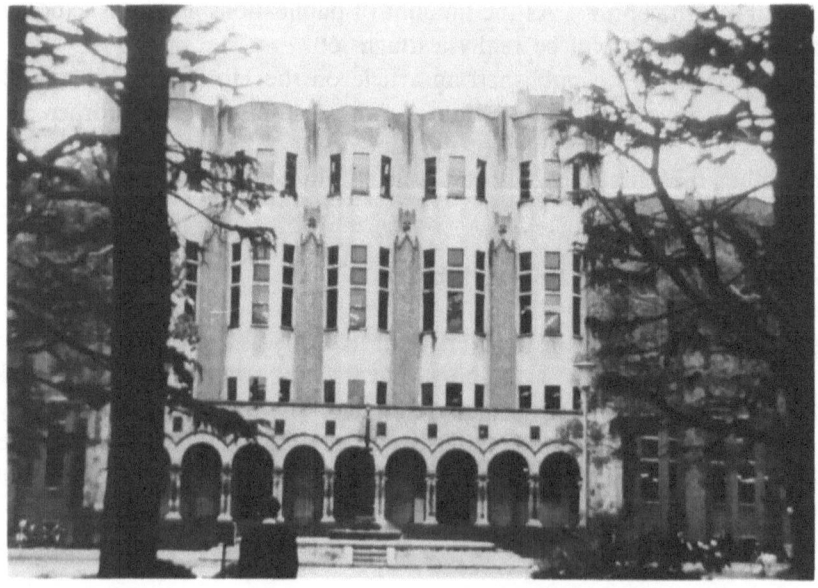

Fig. 1. The entrance of the Central Library (Rockefeller Library) of the University of Tokyo.

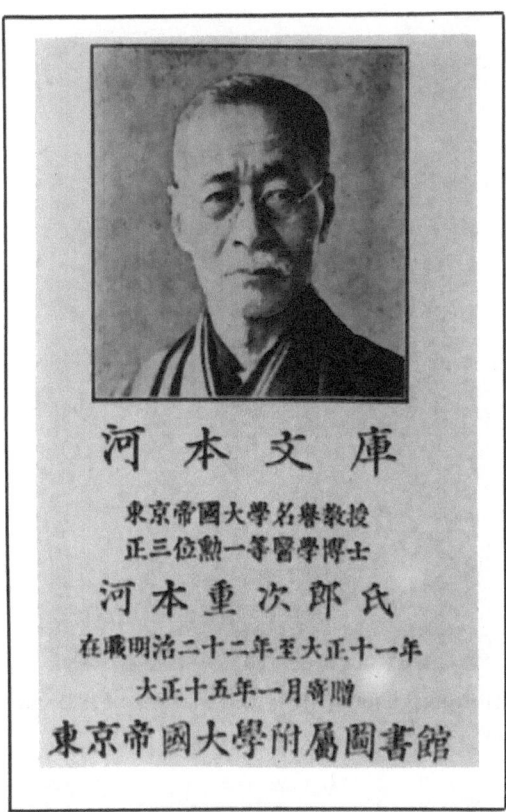

Fig. 2. The label attached to the back of the front cover of books of the Hirschberg Library with Prof. Komoto's portrait. The Japanese characters read from top to bottom: Komoto Library – Prof. Emeritus; Third Rank; First order decoration; doctor of medicine – Komoto Jujiro – professor from 1899 to 1922 – donated in 1926 – Central Library, Imperial University of Tokyo.

buy the library (Fig. 2). It took three years before the library could be shipped to Japan. It was fortunate that the books arrived in Japan after the Tokyo Big Earthquake. The library was donated to the University of Tokyo, to be stored into the newly built Rockefeller Library.

A new catalogue of the Hirschberg Library in Japan was completed in 1939 after three years of hard work and expenses of more than 7000 yen, corresponding to 70 000 US dollars (Fig. 3). This catalogue is composed of four volumes. It has 605 chapters, but the content in the chapters differs considerably from the first edition. On the whole there is now more information stored in the same chapters, as Hirschberg seems to have added material since he published his catalogue in 1901. The library itself now contains over 3000 books and more than 10 000 reprints, many bound together. They are stored in a special room at the 6th floor of the building, numbering from V-650-100 through -1691, occupying three racks with 63 columns (Fig. 4).

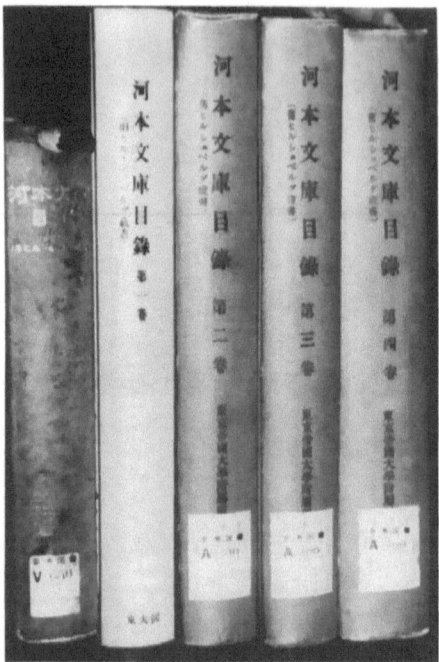

Fig. 3. Index of the Hirschberg Library (left: the first Index of 1901; the four volumes to the right: the Japanese Index of 1939).

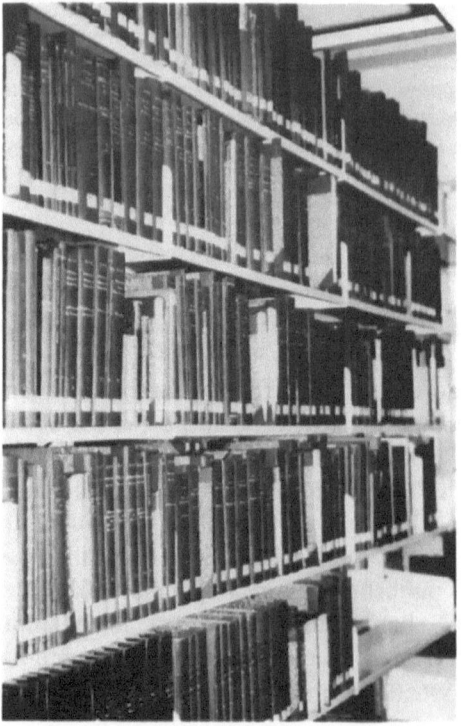

Fig. 4. The Hirschberg Library in the racks.

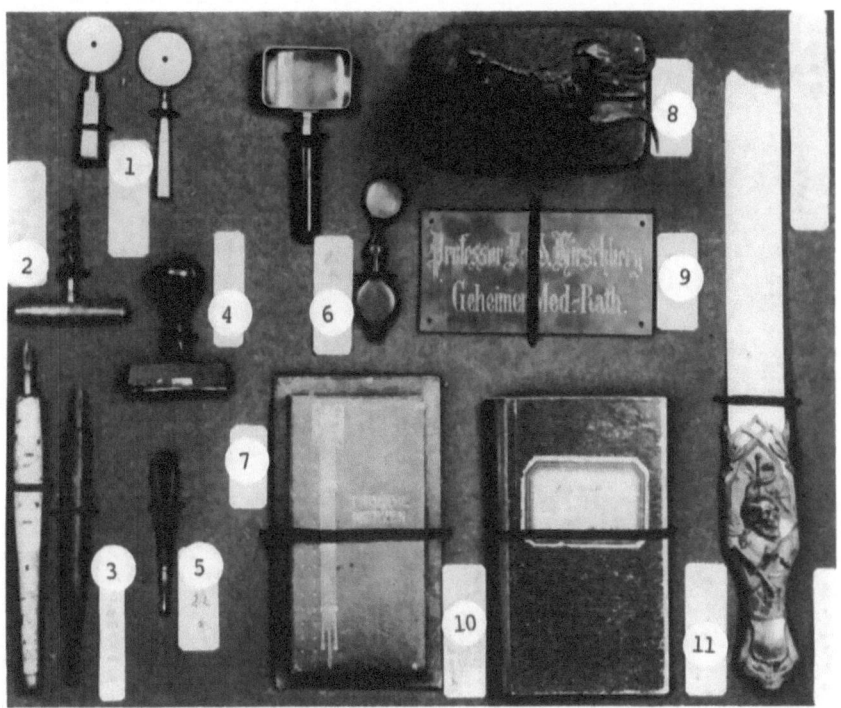

Fig. 5. Instruments used by Hirschberg: (1) mirror for indirect ophthalmoscopy and skiscopy; (2) cork screw; (3) pens; (4) rubber stamp; (5) epilation forceps; (6) loupes; (7) everyday's memobook; (8) penholder; (9) name plate; (10) handwritten diary (1896); (11) paper-knife.

Fifty numbers were missing when I visited the library. Among those missing, thirty were missing in the catalogue itself. Another twelve were located elsewhere in the library. Yet another eight may be somewhere else in the general library, but are hard to trace at present. Some books are stored in other racks under a different classification. But on the whole, the library seems to be stored in good condition.

Hirschberg's ophthalmological instruments (Fig. 5) along with his handwritten diary of 1896 (Fig. 6), were bought by Prof. Shigeru Kagoshima, who looked after the transportation of the Hirschberg Library from Germany to Japan. These objects are now stored at the Alumni Building of Kumamoto University of Medical School where Prof. Kagoshima worked from 1926 to 1941. The objects are in good condition.

Conclusion

Although the Hirschberg Library is used only by a few scholars today, it remains a precious and useful collection of ophthalmic literature, especially

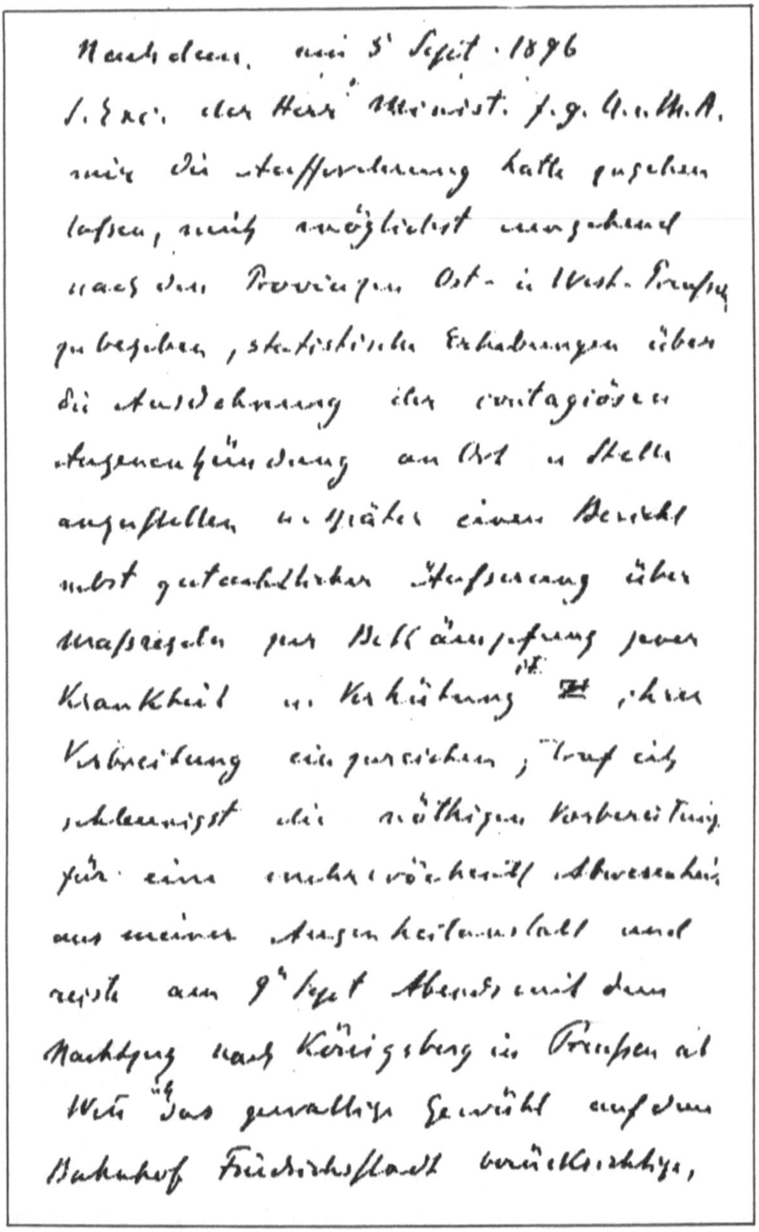
Nachdem am 5. Sept. 1896
S. Exc. der Herr Minist. f. g. U. u. M. A.
mir die Aufforderung hatte zugehen
lassen, mich möglichst umgehend
nach den Provinzen Ost- u. West-Preußen
zu begeben, statistische Erhebungen über
die Ausdehnung der contagiösen
Augenentzündung an Ort u. Stelle
anzustellen u. später einen Bericht
nebst gutachtlicher Äußerung über
Maßregeln zur Bekämpfung jener
Krankheit u. Verhütung ihrer
Verbreitung einzureichen, traf ich
schleunigst die nöthigen Vorbereitungen
für eine mehrwöchentliche Abwesenheit
aus meiner Augenheilanstalt und
reiste am 9. Sept. Abends mit dem
Nachtzug nach Königsberg in Preußen ab.
Was das gewaltige Gewühl auf dem
Bahnhof Friedrichstadt berücksichtige,

Fig. 6. A page of Hirschberg's diary (1896).

as old literature on ophthalmology is scanty in Japan. Recently I read Arthur Hailey's novel *Roots* and I was quite surprised to learn that the records of ships of two hundred years ago are still kept in good order so that the author could trace back the history of the ships by record. Old literature is precious, but as the amount of new information increases exponentially, the method of storing the information is rapidly changing. Computers will be utilized more and more, such as is the case in publishing information on the sequence of DNA and proteins. At the same time, books and journals will continue to be just as important, for the exchange of results and of new ideas, and for reviews.

References

1. Neue Deutsche Biographie, Bd. 9, p. 221.
2. S. Sakai and A. Nakajima: Hirschberg Library, in: Historia Ophthalmologica Internationalis, Vol. 1(2), 1979, pp. 149–155.
3. Y. Ando: A Short History of the Central Library of the University of Tokyo, 1978. Brochure published by the Library commemorating the 50th Anniversary of the restored library.

Address for correspondence: Dr. A. Nakajima, Department of Ophthalmology, Juntendo University, Tokyo 113, Japan.

Documenta Ophthalmologica **81**: 111–119, 1992.
© 1992 *Kluwer Academic Publishers.*

A case of eye disease (Lippitudo) on the Roman frontier in Britain

ANTHONY R. BIRLEY

Düsseldorf, Germany

Key words: History of ophthalmology, eye disease in Roman empire (lippitudo), Roman army, Vindolanda (Britain), writing-tablets

Abstract. A newly excavated Roman report, written in ink on wood, on the strength of the First Cohort of Tungrians at Vindolanda in northern Britain, registers 31 men unfit, 15 as sick, 6 as wounded, the remainder, 10, with eye-disease, 'lippientes'. The paper also comments on the prevalence of eye-disease in antiquity and some of the suggested causes thereof.

Persons with inflamed and swollen eyes, *lippi*, were evidently a common sight in ancient Rome.[1] Since the condition rendered the sufferer unfit for work, but not necessarily confined to bed, *lippi* were bracketed with barbers as purveyors of news or gossip: they could hang about all day exchanging the latest. So, at any rate, the poet Horace put it: 'omnibus et lippis notum et tonsoribus esse'.[2] 'Lippitudo' was clearly an all-purpose term for a variety of minor eye-troubles, caused, the ancients believed, by glaring sunlight, journeys, smoke, dust, massage oil, and irregular habits. Apart from avoidance of direct light, treatment of mild cases seems to have been frequently by means of a salve or ointment. Galen and other medical writers describe such preparations.[3] Further, many hundreds of 'oculists' stamps' have been found, used to impress on the block or stick of ointment, *collyrium*, the name of the doctor or apothecary who prescribed it and particulars of the preparation, e.g. T.ATTI DIVIXTI DIAZMYRNES POST IMP(ETUM) LIP(PITUDINIS) [Titus Attius Divixtus' Diazmyrnes (i.e. myrrh-based) after the onset of inflammation].[4]

For reasons which have not yet been explained virtually all these oculists' stamps have been found in the north-western part of the Roman empire, i.e. in Gaul, Germany and Britain.[5] Certainly, some of the factors the ancients believed to be responsible were especially likely to have affected soldiers along the Rhine and in the army of Britain: long marches, heat, dust and smoke. Galen, in fact, mentions that an oculist, named Axius, attached to the British fleet, *classis Britannica*, based at Boulogne, devised an eye-salve made up of eight different ingredients, including mercuric sulphide.[6] In spite of this concentration of evidence, there is no particular reason to believe that eye-infections were more widespread in the north-western provinces of the Roman empire than in other parts of the ancient world.[7]

For all that, it is perhaps worth registering a new piece of evidence of

112

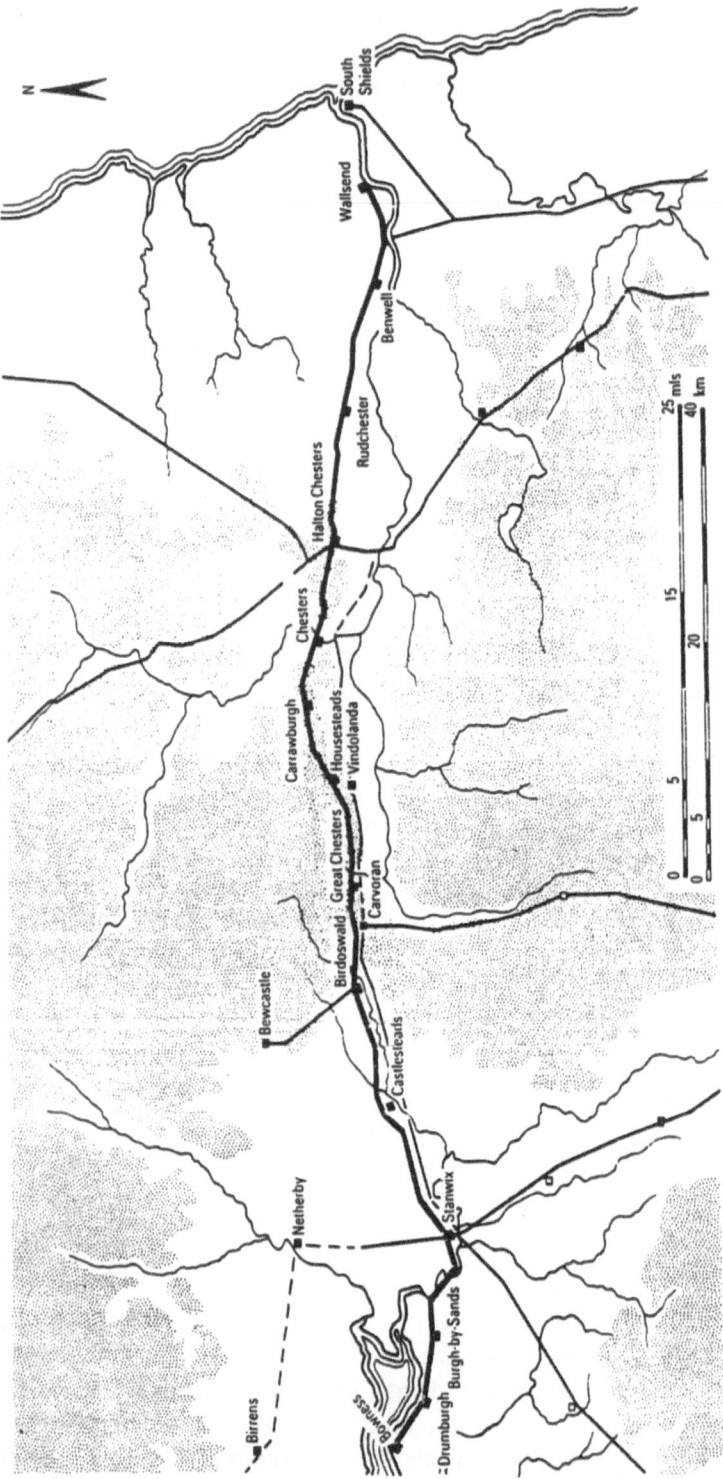

Fig. 1. The Roman frontier in Britain. The dark line is Hadrian's Wall (with kind permission of Dr D.J. Breeze).

'lippitudo' from a fort on the Roman frontier in Britain. It appears, for one thing, to be the first documentary attestation – as opposed to literary – of the word 'lippientes'. On a 'strength report' of the garrison, those unfit for duty are listed in three categories: sick (*aegri*), wounded (*volnerati*), and 'lippientes'.[8]

The site at which this find was made had the Roman – or indeed Celtic – name Vindolanda. It lies approximately one kilometre south of the mid-point of Hadrian's Wall, on the Roman road now known as the Stanegate, and was first constructed in the early 80s of the first century AD, some forty years before Hadrian ordered the construction of the Wall.[9] It was garrisoned by the Roman army continuously until the end of Roman rule in Britain at the beginning of the 5th century AD, with numerous superimposed building periods, creating occupation in places to a depth of more than seven metres below present ground level. Earlier excavations concentrated on the visible stone fort, built in the second century, with several reconstructions thereafter. It was only in the 1970s that the Director of Excavations of the Vindolanda Trust, Robin Birley, was able to detect no fewer than five previous successive timber forts, belonging to the years ca. AD 85–140, that lie beneath the stone fort and camp village (*vicus*) which grew up outside it. What has made these excavations of particular interest and importance is the unusually well-preserved state of the Roman organic material: wood, leather, textiles, vegetation, even pupae of stable-flies, have all been preserved by a combination of damp soil conditions and the seal of puddled clay and other material laid by the Roman military engineers each time they rebuilt. In the anaerobic environment thus created virtually everything seems to have survived.[10]

Of all these finds there can be no question that the most valuable have been the so-called 'writing-tablets', thin slices of wood, mostly alder and birch, shaped and prepared, on which letters and records were written in ink. It had always been known that the Roman army, like modern armies, generated mounds of paper. But papyrus, the standard equivalent of paper in the ancient world, has not survived in western military sites. Only Egypt and Syria have preserved Roman military records on this material, which was in any case no doubt too expensive for daily use in the west.[11] There, it was assumed, the army used wooden writing tablets spread with wax in a recess, written on with a metal stylus. They could be used and re-used several times, which creates a major problem for modern archaeologists when they survive. Assuming that the writer scratched through the wax and left traces, there is generally a jumble of successive texts. This kind of writing-tablet has been frequently found and was in use at Vindolanda too. But the excavations by Robin Birley have produced over a thousand examples of the thin 'leaf-tablet' written on with ink, previously unknown. Since a good many are letters sent to Vindolanda from elsewhere, they were clearly used throughout the Roman army in Britain.[12]

Many are mere scraps or fragments, but several supply fascinating detail

Fig. 2. 'Writing-tablet' from Vindolanda, ca. AD 90. The word 'lippientes' occurs in the 2nd line from the bottom (photograph by Alison Rutherford).

on daily life and military routine of a remote Roman frontier post. One delightful example is a letter from a woman called Claudia Severa, inviting her 'dearest sister, my soul', Sulpicia Lepidina, to come to her birthday party. Lepidina was the wife of the Vindolanda commandant, Flavius Cerialis, prefect of the Ninth Cohort of Batavians, Claudia Severa's husband was Aelius Brocchus, another Roman officer, stationed at one of the other

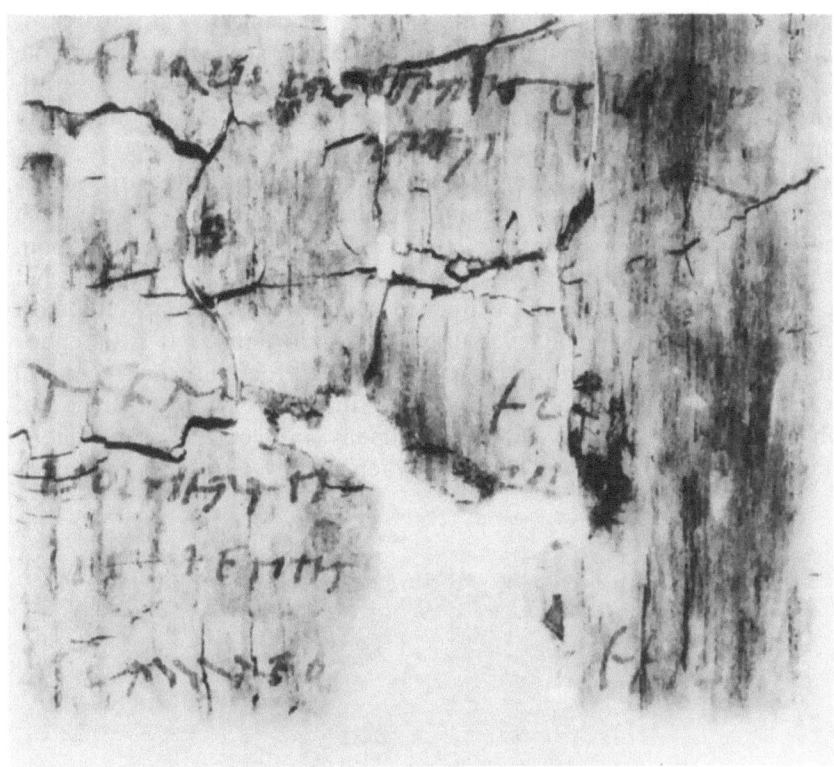

Fig. 3. Detail of fig. 2 (photograph by Alison Rutherford).

frontier forts. A letter was sent to Vindolanda from London by a man called Chrauttius – a Germanic name, suggesting that he was a former member of the Batavian regiment – to his 'brother' Veldedeius, the governor's groom, demanding news, sending greetings, and adding a firm message for Virilis, the *veterinarius*, to send 'by one of our people' the shears he had promised to sell.[13] The largest number of letters and documents do indeed derive from the period, ca. AD 100, when the Batavians were based at Vindolanda.

The Batavians, a Germanic people living in what is now the Netherlands, where the Betuwe area perpetuates their name, were a major supplier of 'auxiliary' troops to the Roman army. Eight of their regiments served in Britain from the conquest in AD 43 and – after reorganisation following their mutiny and revolt in AD 69–70 – at least four were back in Britain in the period of further Roman expansion in Britain that began in the 70s.[14] Tacitus mentions 'four cohorts of Batavians and two of Tungrians' as fighting for Rome against the Caledonians at the battle of Mons Graupius in AD 83.[15] The Ninth Batavians came to Vindolanda some years later, rebuilding the first fort there. They were to leave, presumably then commanded by Flavius Cerialis, in AD 102, first to serve in what is now

Rumania, then in Bavaria, where they gave their name to Castra Batava-Passau.[16] Their predecessor and successor as garrison at Vindolanda was the First Cohort of Tungrians. The Tungrians, another Germanic people, with considerable Celtic elements, had their centre at the modern Tongeren in Belgium.[17]

Identification of the First Tungrians as Vindolanda's original garrison was made possible by the finding of an unusually large writing-tablet in the ditch of the earliest fort. Exceptionally, it was of oak, measuring 39.4 × 8.6 cm, carrying a text of 27 lines. Parts of the text are now lost or illegible, but what remains is enough for the editors to describe it as perhaps 'the most important military document ever discovered in Britain'.[18] It is a report, dated 18 May in an unknown year – assignable from the archaeological context to ca. AD 90 – of the 'net number of the First Cohort of Tungrians, of which the commander is Julius Verecundus, prefect: 752 men, among them centurions, 6.' Well over half the soldiers and five out of six centurions

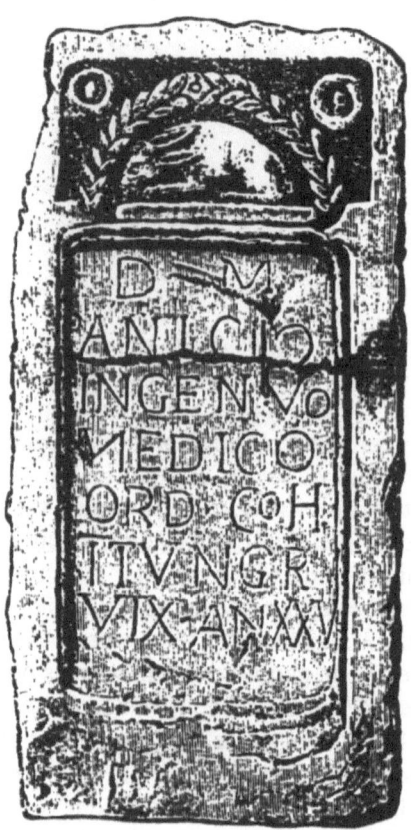

Fig. 4. Tombstone from Housesteads on Hadrian's Wall: D.M. Anicio Ingenuo medico ord. coh. I Tungr. vix. an. XXV [To the divine shades (and) Anicius Ingenuus, medicus ordinarius of the First Cohort of Tungrians, lived 25 years] (with kind permission of Dr D.J. Breeze).

were registered as absent, seconded for various duties elsewhere, for example 46 men on the headquarters staff of an officer called Ferox, perhaps a legionary commander; one centurion, if that is the correct reading, was at London; and a large group of men were at 'Coris', probably Corbridge-on-Tyne, a major frontier base. Of the 296 men actually at Vindolanda, 'reliqui praesentes', 31 were listed as unfit:

aegri	xv	sick	15
volnerati	vi	wounded	6
lippientes	[x]	with eye-trouble	[10]
summa eo[rum]	xxxi	total of these	31[19]

No doubt the First Cohort of Tungrians had at least one medical orderly or doctor in their ranks. As it happens, a tombstone from the nearby Hadrian's Wall fort of Housesteads commemorates a later 'medicus ord(inarius)' of the regiment, Anicius Ingenuus, who died at the age of 25.[20] At Vindolanda, a few years after Julius Verecundus' report on the Tungrians was compiled, there was a 'medicus' with the Batavians, registered as accompanying a building-party.[21] This was a prudent practice, paralleled by inscriptions of legionary working parties from Iversheim in Germany[22] and Almus in Bulgaria.[23] Soldiers were as likely to be injured in peace-time activity as to be wounded in warfare. No trace of eye-salves has yet been found at Vindolanda, but a leather eye-patch unearthed in the excavations of 1991 was more probably worn by a sufferer from 'lippitudo' than by a man who had lost his eye in battle.

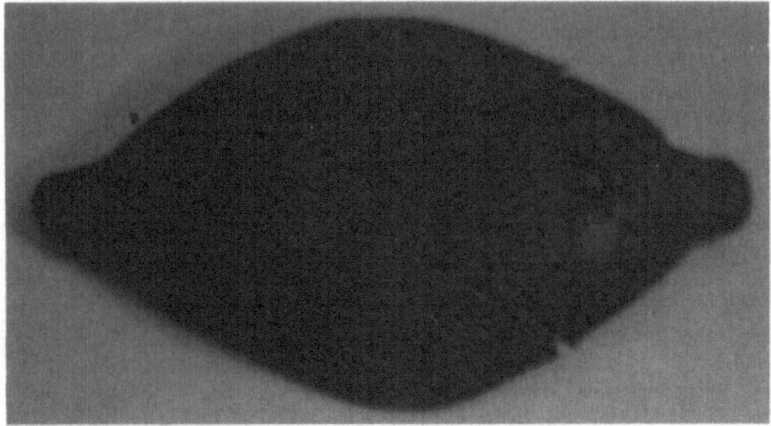

Fig. 5. Roman eye patch, made of leather, found in the excavations at Vindolanda in 1991, in a second century AD level. Dimensions: 95 mm × 50 mm; average thickness of leather is 2.8 mm.

118

Notes

1. A useful summary account is provided by Kind, Real-Encyclopädie der classischen Altertumswissenschaft XIII/1, 1926, cols. 723–6, art. 'Lippitudo'. Cf. now R. Jackson, Doctors and Diseases in the Roman Empire, London 1988, 82 ff.
2. Horace, Satires I.7,3.
3. E.g. Galen XII p. 725 Kühn; Celsus, De Med. VI 6,1. The Elder Pliny mentions the condition and treatments for it in various places in his Natural History.
4. Corpus Inscriptionum Latinarum III 1636 = XIII 10021, 19 = H. Dessau, Inscriptiones Latinae Selectae, Berlin 1892–1916, 8737.
5. See above all the thorough study by G.C. Boon, 'Potters, oculists and eye-troubles', Britannia XIV, 1983, 1–12. He notes, p. 3 f., that at the end of 1977 a total of 240 provenanced examples were known, only one of which came from outside Europe (Numidia).
6. Galen XII p. 786 Kühn (who misunderstood the text). Boon, op. cit. 6 n. 32, notes that 'Axios is a common name'. One should also recall that 'Axius' was a Roman family name, cf. e.g. Quintus Axius, the friend of Varro (De re rustica III 2,1). But it must be conceded that doctors in the Roman world were frequently Greeks, or had Greek names.
7. Boon, op. cit. 4 f., no doubt rightly regards the ancient explanations – marches, smoke, dust etc. (Marcellus Empiricus, De Medicamentis VIII, p. 121 Liechtenhan) – as inadequate. As he himself shows, 10 ff. deficiencies in diet, particularly lack of greenstuffs and fruit, and in hygiene, were the basic cause. As for the distribution of oculists' stamps, he concludes that 'in the south and east [of the Roman empire] there were probably more doctors, and medicines were probably more often expressly compounded. In that case they would not need so permanent a marking, only a label on their box, jar or bottle', p. 9.
8. The Thesaurus Linguae Latinae VII 2 ii, Leipzig 1970–1979, cols. 1472 f., gives no example of the word from any inscription (other than oculists' stamps) or papyrus. The new document is published by A.K. Bowman and J.D. Thomas, 'A military strength report from Vindolanda', Journal of Roman Studies LXXXI, 1991, 62–73.
9. R. Birley, Vindolanda. A Roman frontier post on Hadrian's Wall, London 1977, reports on the excavations up to 1975.
10. R. Birley, op. cit., 103 ff. A full report on the excavations up to 1989 by the same author, Vindolanda, The Early Wooden Forts, is at the press (London, English Heritage).
11. R.O. Fink, Roman Military Records on Papyrus, Cleveland 1971.
12. The examples found in the 1970s were published by A.K. Bowman and J.D. Thomas, Vindolanda: the Latin Writing-Tablets, Britannia Monograph Series no. 4, London 1983. For later finds, n. 8, above, and n. 13.
13. A.K. Bowman and J.D. Thomas, 'New texts from Vindolanda', Britannia XVIII, 1987, 125–142, at pp. 137–140; eid., with J.N. Adams, 'Two letters from Vindolanda', ibid. XXI, 1990, 33–52, at pp. 33–41.
14. K. Strobel, 'Anmerkungen zur Geschichte der Bataverkohorten in der hohen Kaiserzeit', Zeitschrift für Papyrologie und Epigraphik LXX, 1987, 271–292, was able to incorporate some of the new information from Vindolanda.
15. Tacitus, Agricola 36,1.
16. A.R. Birley, 'Vindolanda: notes on some new writing tablets', Zeitschrift f. Pap. u. Epigr. LXXXI, 1991, 87–102, at p. 87, with n. 3; Strobel, op. cit. (n. 14 above).
17. E.M. Wightman, Gallia Belgica, London 1985, 53 f., etc.
18. Bowman and Thomas, op. cit. (n. 8 above) 62.
19. The editors very properly print the first four letters of 'lippientes' with dots underneath: 'palaeographically, the reading of the first four letters is unclear but the traces are compatible with the reading suggested'. The present writer was able to read 'lippientes' independently, from study of the photographs and of the writing-tablet itself, before publication of the text.

20. R.G. Collingwood and R.P. Wright, The Roman Inscriptions of Britain, I, Oxford 1965, p. 1618. On this question, see R.W. Davies, 'The Roman military medical service', Saalburg-Jahrbuch XXVII, 1970, 84–104, reprinted in his posthumously published Service in the Roman Army, ed. D. Breeze and V.A. Maxfield, Edinburgh 1989, 209 ff.
21. Unpublished, Inventory no. 248.
22. Corpus Inscriptionum Latinarum XIII 7943 (AD 145).
23. Ibid. III 7449 (AD 155).

Address for correspondence: Prof. Dr Anthony R. Birley, Heinrich-Heine Universität Düsseldorf, Abt. Alte Geschichte, Historisches Seminar, Universitätsstrasse 1, Gebäude 23.31.05, W-4000 Düsseldorf 1, Germany.

Documenta Ophthalmologica **81**: 121–132, 1992.
© 1992 *Kluwer Academic Publishers*.

Some Byzantine chroniclers and historians on ophthalmological topics

JOHN FRONIMOPOULOS & JOHN LASCARATOS
Athens, Greece

Key words: History of ophthalmology, Byzantium

Abstract. Byzantine historians and chroniclers recorded events not only of national importance, but also of daily life. The authors present various aspects in relation to ophthalmology. A selection of subjects including eye disorders and injuries, as well as visual problems discussed in myths, narratives and religious dogmas are presented.

Introduction

In the history of Byzantium, the texts written by the historians and the chroniclers are of great importance. The historians relating and researching social, national and important historical events, wrote with objectivity and culture, without phantasy, using the official language. On the other hand the chroniclers recorded events from daily life, without any literary pretention or interpretations of the facts. As most of the chroniclers originated from monasteries, they sought to arouse the interest of the public in the beliefs and dogmas of the Orthodox Christian Church.

From the texts of these historians and chroniclers we have gathered information which gives us a general view of the spirit of the age in regard to how ophthalmological topics were perceived. The information fluctuates between actual events and narratives from the realm of myth, prejudice and even religious dogma and has been grouped according to subject matter.

1. Teratogenesis

Georgios Cedrenos, the chronicler (11th century), describes in his writings [3] the following cases of teratogenesis. (1) During the time of Theodosius, son of Maurice, (582–602 AD), a woman in Daonion gave birth to a child that neither had eyes or eyelids, nor hands or feet. In the hip region there was a fish-tail covered with scales. We regard this as a case of anophthalmia, ablepharia, in a monster with ichthyasis. On the same day a dog with six feet and a head resembling a lion was also born. (2) In Antioch, a child was born in perfect physical condition, except for a single eye in the middle of its forehead. It also had four hands and four feet and a chin. We regard this as a case of a cyclops.

The chronicler *Ioannis Curopalates* mentions that during the reign of Ioannis Cantacuzenus (1347–1354, Skylitzes, 11th century) a child was born in Constantinople with a single eye in its forehead and the legs of a goat. Similarly he notes the birth of a hen with three legs [5]. Another chronicler, *Theophanes* (8th–9th century) mentions the birth of a child without eyes, eyelids, hands or feet. It had a fish tail attached to its hip [16]. Clearly this refers to the same case mentioned above by *Georgios Cedrenos* [3].

The chronicler *Zonaras* (11th–12th century) mentions the same case with the following description: '... and then the sun grew dark and a woman in Thrace gave birth to a child without eyes or eyelids, hands or feet and with a fishtail attached to its hip [7]'. The historian *Michael Attaleiates* (11th century) also mentions this case which he describes as follows: 'During the same year some monsters were born in the city of Byzas. A child with a single eye in the centre of its forehead was born. It had the feet of a goat. A hen with three legs was also born' [10].

2. Gelimerus' eye disease

The historian *Procopius* (6th century) mentions the eye disease of Gelimerus, King of Goths, reigning from 530–534 AD (Fig. 1). In this disease one eye had swollen due to uncleanness and it was for this reason

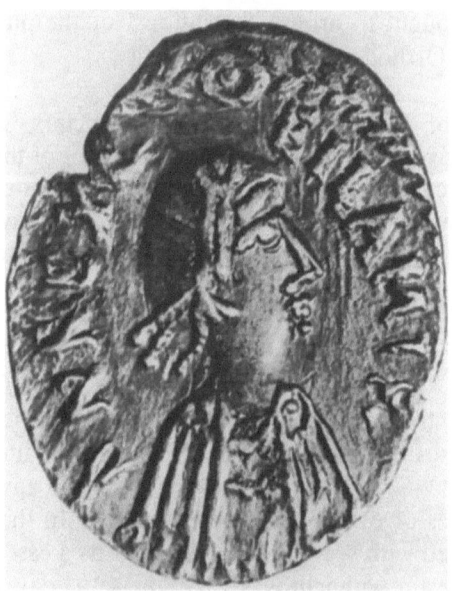

Fig. 1. Gelimerus, King of Goths (silver coin).

that he was obliged to use a sponge to clean it. The historian stresses that cleanness is indispensable for the health of the eyes [15].

3. Photophobia

Regarding photophobia, the historian *Ioannis Cantacuzenos* (14th century) mentions that '. . . it is difficult for those suffering from ophthalmia to look into the sun, while darkness is more comfortable for them [6]. In the dark it is also pleasant for them to blink because they cannot easily bear the light' (Fig. 2).

4. Eyelid trauma

The historian *Leo the Deacon* (10th century) refers to the injury of the eyelid of Bardas, son of the emperor Nicephorus Phocas (963–969 AD, Fig. 3). This wound constituted one of the reasons for Nicephorus' abdication

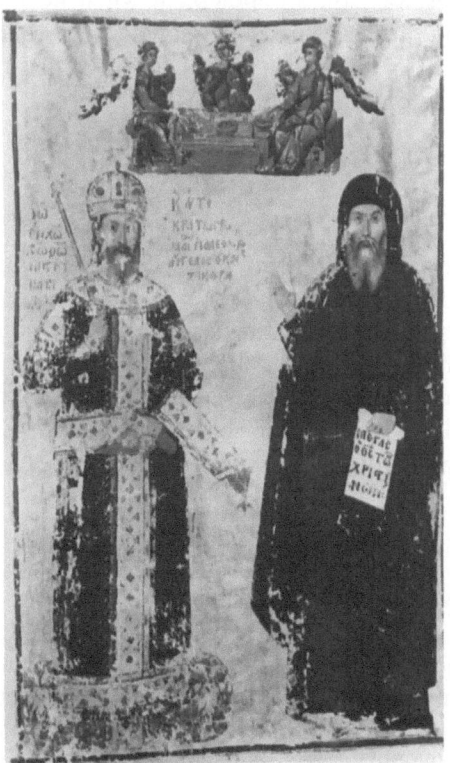

Fig. 2. Ioannis Cantacuzinos as emperor and monk (National Library of Paris).

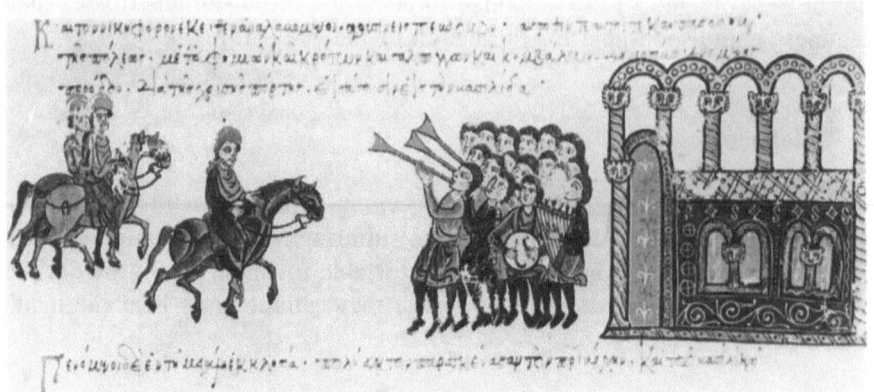

Fig. 3. The emperor Nicephorus Phocas' triumphal entry into Constantinople (Chronicler Scylitzes, National Library, Madrid, Spain).

from the throne which he ceded to Ioannis Tsimisces. Regarding this he writes: '. . . he (Phocas) did not originally accept the authority, frightened by the envy which accompanies the acquisition of such a high estate and excused himself on the grounds of the death of his wife as well as that of his son, Bardas. Bardas was still an adolescent when he was wounded by his nephew, Pleusis, due to a spear which pierced the eyelid. It was a serious wound and the point of the spear passed through the cranium and Bardas fell from his horse, stone dead' [9].

5. The perception of colour

The historian *Nicephorus Gregoras* (14th century) makes noteworthy remarks regarding the perception of colour [13]. He maintained that intellect ('nous') is what perceives and distinguishes various colours, just as each of us can perceive through our senses the various textures of objects. Through the sense of touch we perceive, via the intellect, the roughness and smoothness of bodies. Through the sense of smell we perceive the fragrant and foul odours and through the sense of hearing we perceive harmonious sounds.

6. Proptosis of the eyeball; exophthalmos

The historian *Procopius* (6th century) mentions a characteristic case of exophthalmos during the torture of one Theodoros Diogenes by the empress Theodora [15]. At first, he mentions, they used fair means but because these brought no result, Theodora ordered that his head be bound by a cowhide whip. It was tied about his ears and twisted tighter and tighter. The historian writes that Theodora expected the eyeballs to be pressed out of their sockets.

7. Strabismus

The historian *Nicephorus Gregoras* (14th century) mentions St. Gregory Palamas (1296–1359 AD, Fig. 4) in a discussion he had with certain pneumatomachoi (enemies of the Holy Spirt) as follows: '. . . Those who leave our country in a bad manner, quarrel amongst themselves like cross-eyes, each of which looks at a thing (image) separately and grows distant from its correct place, a malady called squinting but not blindness' [13]. Another historian, *Georgios Pachymeres*, (13th century AD, Fig. 5) writes that the Patriarch Vekkos, addressing the Emperor Michael VIII (1259–1282 AD, Fig. 6) requests his clemency for certain people he characterizes as suffering from strabismus [4].

The chronicler Ducas (15th century AD) describes the eyes of Andronicus IV (1376–1379) and Ioannis VII (1390), writing that Andronicus had one staring eye, very widely open, and that Ioannis, his son, had eyes both of

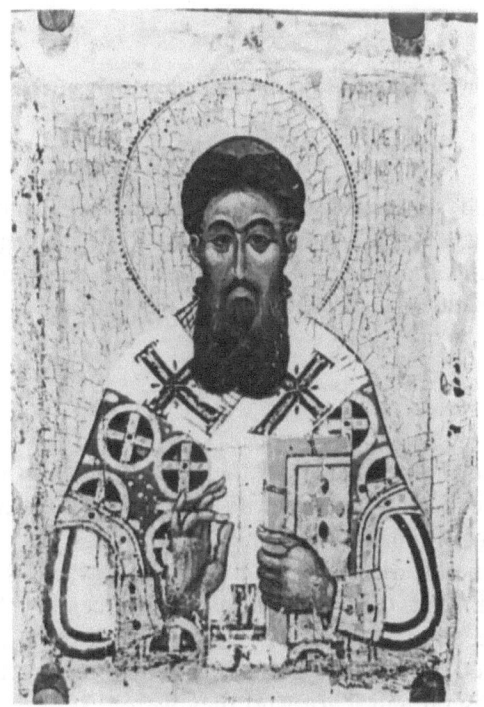

Fig. 4. St. Gregory Palamas (icon of the 15th century, Museum of Fine Arts, St. Petersburg, Russia).

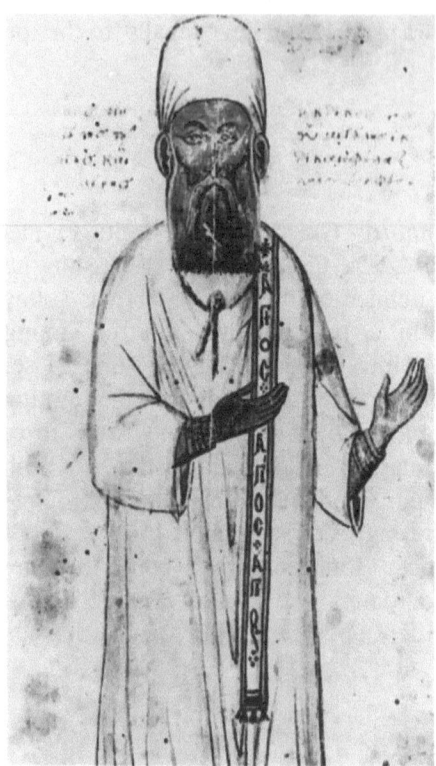

Fig. 5. Georgios Pachymeres (manuscript of the 14th century, Bavarian National Library, Munich, Germany).

which blinked and stared as well as squinted [11]. Another chronicler, *Constantine Manasses* (12th century AD), when describing Ioannis Tzimisces (969–976) writes that the latter had a lowered glance or gaze (hamiloblepharon) and a pleasing expression [1].

8. Amblyopia

The historians and the chroniclers of the period used the term a amblyopia to indicate the weakening of sight with age. *Michael Glycas* (12th century AD [12]) mentions a similar occurrence which takes place when the snake grows very old. Then it will suffer from amblyopia which is accompanied by abstaining from all food. *Georgios Cedrenus* (11th century AD) [3], uses the term varyopia instead of the term amblyopia. He mentions that '... the eyes of Israel, weakened by age, see dimly but in spite of this they managed to see the sons of Joseph and learn who they were'.

The same chronicler also uses the term amblyopia to mean a weakening of vision in old age, and describes a mythological event: '... When Perseus

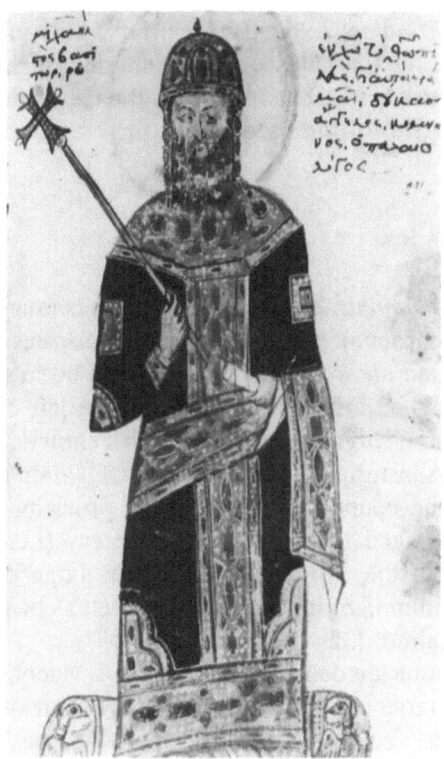

Fig. 6. Emperor Michael VIII (manuscript of the 14th century, Bavarian National Library, Munich, Germany).

came out he was displaying the head of the Gorgon. He did not know that Kipheas had dim vision due to age, but as he approached him on horseback he realised that the Gorgon's head he was holding did not have the usual effect. Then he turned the head towards himself and facing it, he was instantly blinded'.

9. Vision at night; interpretation of vision

(1) The chronicler *Michael Glycas* (12th century AD) [12] interprets the vision of animals which circulate at night as follows: 'If you look for the reasons why felines and bats see so well at night, these reasons are to be found in the very delicate visual spirit. This spirit expands slightly during the night due to the absence of the sun and thus becomes capable of perceiving objects. Conversely during the day, due to the great delicacy of the visual spirit, the ability to see is diminished. This same phenomenon is observed in lions which avoid solar reflections throughout the length of the day and hide from the sun's rays. If this were not the case and they could walk about unhindered, they would see and attack animals or people' [12].

(2) The historian *Ioannis Lydos* (6th century AD) in his manuscript *de Mensibus* writes that the ibis can see only on moonlit nights: 'On a moonless night the ibis cannot see, so these birds shut their eyes during this time and fast, awaiting the arrival of the moonlight' [8].

10. Anomalies of the iris

(1) The chronicler *Ioannis Zonaras'* (11th–12th century AD) referring to the dikoria (heterochromia) of the emperor Anastasius (491–518) writes: 'Anastasius was named *dikoros* (having two irises) because his irises did not match. The right iris had a darker colour than the left one [7].

(2) The chronicler *Georgios Cedrenus* (11th century AD) also refers to this description of Anastasius' eyes, writing that, 'after the death of Zeno (491), the queen, the council and the armies proclaim Anastasius Selentiarius king. He belonged to the acephalon heresy (i.e., the unconverted Monophysites) that is the Synchytikon. He was large of stature and had happy eyes of a medium light hue (glaucos) as well as being a little bald and he was also white-haired' [3].

(3) The same chronicler describes the eyes of Valentinianus (364–378), writing that 'he was large of stature and florid in colour of the skin. His hair was fair and his eyes were handsome and tended to be light-coloured' [3].

11. The expression of feelings – tears

(1) The historian *Theophylactus Simocatta* (6th–7th century AD) referring to the death of King Maurice (582–602) wrote: 'This sorrowful event was so deeply felt that many people wept so much that their tears resembled a flooding river. Indeed his death provoked rivers of tears and many of his subjects mourned deeply' [17].

(2) The historian *Michael Attaleiates* (11th century AD) referring to the pitiful fate of the blinded Emperor Romanus IV Diogenes (1065–1071), writes that he had 'dissolved his eyes and face with a rain of tears' [10].

(3) The chronicler *Ioannis Zonaras* (11th–12th century AD) writes that 'when Basilios II (976–1025) saw how humbled the mighty usurper Bardas Sclerus became, when in his last years he was old and blind and was to be led by the hand, he instantly turned his eyes away from sheer sorrow' [7].

12. Bloodstained tears

Nicetas Choniates (12th–13th century AD, Fig. 7) referring to scenes from the conquest of Constantinople by the Crusaders of the Fourth Crusade

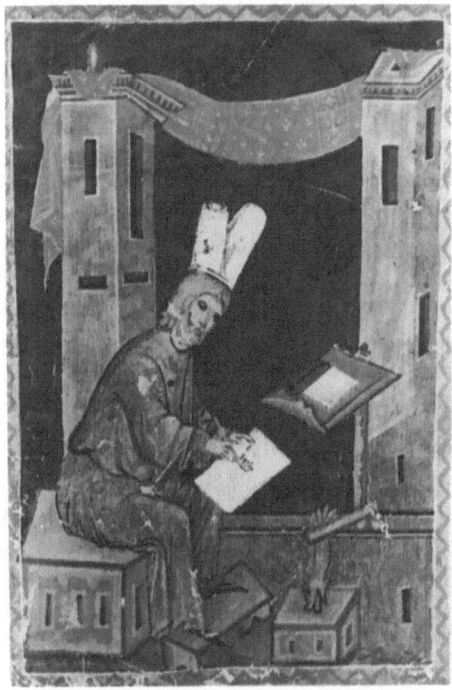

Fig. 7. Nicetas Choniates (manuscript of the 14th century, National Library, Vienna, Austria).

(1204) writes about the soldiers that 'they had lost their colour and had an aspect similar to that of dead men. Their eyes were bloodshot for they shed more blood than tears' [14].

13. Optic phenomena

Michael Glycas (12th century AD) referring to the rainbow writes that 'there is no rainbow in reality; it is only an illusion of vision. This illusion is created when the sun falls on irregular clouds. In this manner the halo about the moon is also an optical illusion' [12].

14. Folklore and prejudice

(1) The chronicler *Michael Glycas* (12th century AD) writes that 'a bird of prey (charadrios) will close its eyes if it looks by chance at someone suffering from jaundice. The bird does not do this, as some say, to avoid hexing the sufferer with the evil eye or conversely to cure him, but in order to avoid becoming infected by this contagious disease' [12].

(2) The same chronicler, referring to mythical dragons says that 'flames

shoot forth from their eyes and the venom they vomit or spit forth is smoky and tears to pieces whomever it touches' [12].

(3) He goes on to mention that the basilisk kills with its glance alone anyone who lays eyes on it. And the Holy Scripture mentions that this reptile can turn the evil eye on a man. Experience and time have shown, from older times, as this author writes, that 'the eyes act as well as sufferer, sometimes emitting signals and at other-moments receiving signals as happens with the eyes of lovers' [12]. He further mentions the opinion of Basil the Great (33rd Psalm) who maintains that 'poisoned arrows or darts shoot forth from the eyes (he means from the evil eye) is unacceptable to him, because it is a popular and accepted belief in the quarters of old women' [12].

(4) The historian *Ioannis Lydos* (6th century AD) comments on the curious qualities of the broad bean which in our opinion are related to the beliefs of Pythagoras and other ancient Greek writers. The qualities are related of course to a disorder called kyamismos. The author writes: 'The broad bean (kyamos) which is dedicated to god Ares produces blood in the human system. Men should anoint each other's eyes with a substance extracted from the bean and in this manner should honour Ares' [8].

15. Therapy of those born blind

Michael Glycas (12th century AD) mentions a myth according to which Mary Magdalen met Galen, the doctor. She told him that Christ cured a man blind from birth. Gallen replied to her: 'Then Christ must have studied the metals of the earth for if he had not, he could not make the blind see' [12]. The author classifies this rumour as a myth because he considers it impossible for Mary Magdalen to have met Galen.

16. Vision

The historian *Nicephorus Gregoras* (14th century AD) referring to disorders of vision suffered by drunkards writes in regard to the armies that, 'due to fear, the soldiers suffer from the same disorder as those drunk with wine, i.e. they do not see things naturally or as they are, but in another way. Their vision fluctuates due to the large amount of fluid in the brain so that things in the field of vision appear to be swimming' [13].

17. Similarities and resemblances

Byzantine chroniclers and historians often refer to similarities which are related to vision and its function. *Nicephorus Gregoras* (14th century AD) when facing the heretical doctrines of the Calabrian monk, Varlaam (1290–1350) regarding acts of God, writes that 'St. Paul agrees with his (Gregoras's) view saying that we presently see through a mirror vaguely while later we will see clearly and face to face' [13].

Eunapius (4th century AD) the historian, writes that 'As the light from a candle disappears or grows dull before the rays of the sun, in the same way we shall set truth against what has been said' [2].

Nicephorus Gregoras (14th century AD), writing about the enemies of faith, mentions that 'St. Gregory Palamas, knowing that, just as owls and bats are harmed by the sun which proves convincingly that their eyes are weak, the shaky and rotten doctrines (of the enemies of faith) would be harmed rather than helped by an open discussion in the presence of people'. According to him 'it was preferable that the opponents be crushed by persecutions and punishments, using excuses such as those used in the past by Julian and his followers' [13].

The same author also writes about the Calabrian monk Varlaam, founder of the heresy that Gregoras fought: '. . . and it seems to me he suffered from that mythical lamia (ogress or demon) which was said to live blindly within the house for she had no eyes. But when she came out of her house, she would suddenly acquire eyes which could see so that she could follow all the actions of others with accuracy' [13].

17. The penalty of blinding

Many historians and chroniclers mention the punishment of blinding in Byzantium in 705 AD during the second accession to the throne by the Emperor Justinian II Rhinotmitus (705–711). Among these chroniclers and historians we mention here *Cedrenus*, *Nicephorus*, *Glycas* and others. J. Lascaratos and S. Marketos present information on this subject in this issue [18]. They conclude that this penalty was enforced by various means: (a) by destroying or enucleating the eyes with a sharp instrument, (b) by a fire held close to the eyes, and (c) by pouring a boiling liquid upon the eyes. The writers investigate the grounds for the imposition of the penalty and the methods employed. A series of examples are given as handed down by Byzantine chroniclers.

Conclusion

It is evident that the Byzantine historians and chroniclers provide us with interesting information on ophthalmological topics in relation not only to actual events but also to myths, narratives and religious dogmas. This information gives a picture of the ideas prevalent during the period in Byzantium and shows the influence of ancient beliefs on ophthalmological topics preserved even in Byzantine medicine. However, Byzantine medicine, as a keeper of the Hippocratic, Alexandrian and Galenic teachings, influenced by the Christian spirt of humanism, succeeded in transferring these teachings to Europe, thus contributing essentially to the development of medicine during the Renaissance period.

Bibliography

The 17 references of the authors correspond to the volumes of the historical classical book: Corpus Scriptorum Historiae Byzantinae, editio emendatior et copiosior, consilio B.G. Niebuhrii C.F. (50 volumes Bonnae, E. Weber: 1828–1897).
1. Constantini Manassis: Vol. 29, p. 251.
2. Eunapious: vol. 14, p. 76.
3. Georgius Cedrenos: Vol. 34, p. 41, 68, 548, 625.
4. Georgius Pachymeres: Vol. 24, p. 83, 110, 115, 404, 440.
5. Ioannis Curopalatae: Vol. 35, p. 724.
6. Ioannis Catacuzenus: Vol. 3, p. 434.
7. Ioannis Zonaras: Vol. 45, p. 133, 190, 550.
8. Ioannis Ludi de Mensibus: vol. 31, p. 35, 68.
9. Leon Diaconus: vol 5, p. 21, 40.
10. Michaelis Attaliotae: Vol. 49, p. 177, 211.
11. Michaelis Ducae Nepotis: Vol. 21, p. 46.
12. Michaelis Glycas: Vol. 27, p. 83, 109, 110, 416, 430.
13. Nicephorus Gregoras: Vol. 6, p. 206.
14. Nicetas Choniata de Manuele Comneno: Vol. 23, p. 776.
15. Procopius de Bello Vandalico: Vol. 18, 437; Vol. 28, p. 100.
16. Theophanes: Vol 41, p. 413.
17. Theophylactus Simocata: Vol. 22, p. 37.
18. Lascaratos J., Marketos S.: The penalty of blinding during Byzantine times: Medical remarks. *Documenta Ophthalmologica* 81 (1992): 133–144. History of Ophthalmology, Vol. 5, 1992.

Address for correspondence: Prof. John Fronimopoulos, 6 Neofyton Vambva Street, 10674 Athens, Greece.

Documenta Ophthalmologica **81**: 133–144, 1992.
© 1992 *Kluwer Academic Publishers*.

The penalty of blinding during Byzantine times
Medical remarks

JOHN LASCARATOS & S. MARKETOS
Department of the History of Medicine, Athens University

Key words: History of ophthalmology, purposeful blinding, Byzantium

Abstract. This paper which is based on the works of Byzantine chroniclers examines the imposition of blinding as a penalty in Byzantium. Punishment by blinding, though of extremely ancient origin, was imposed on Christians in the Roman Empire under the rule of Diocletian (AD 303). This continued up to the time of Constantine the Great and blinding as a penalty reappeared in the Byzantine Empire (AD 705) under the rule of Justinian Rhinotmitos. The writers investigate the grounds for the imposition of the penalty, and the methods employed, and a series of examples are given as handed down by Byzantine chroniclers. Finally, the ethical background of the penalty is examined according to the legislature and common-law extant in Byzantium.

The penalty of blinding first appears in Byzantium in 705 AD during the second accession to the throne by Justinian II, the Rhinotmitos. The first victim of this penalty, as mentioned by many chroniclers, was Kallinikos, the Patriarch of Constantinople. As Georgius Cedrenus aptly remarks, 'As he (Justinian II) blinded him, so he banished him to Rome' (Cedrenus 781, 3–4; see also Theophanes 574, 12–13; Grammaticus 169, 3–4; Nicephorus 777, 7, Glycas 518, 14–16; Vasiliev 1932).

It is known for certain, that this penalty was particularly favoured by the Roman emperors who enforced it widely to punish Christians. Its enforcement began with Diocletian in 303 AD and was continued until the reign of Constantine the Great, who ordered its cessation. The history of the penalty, however, is even more ancient because, it appears, it was known and widely enforced by the Eastern races, chiefly in Persia from where it found its way to Byzantium (Lampsidis 1949).

This penalty was suffered by those found guilty of high treason, those practising oracular arts, captives, and whoever belonged to the vanquished side in the religious controversies that riddled the Byzantium of the Icono-clasts, but mainly by conspirators, insurgents and above all *leaders* of revolts against Byzantine emperors, or further those suspected of such a crime. The Byzantine chroniclers and historians also mention a considerable number of emperors who were blinded in cases where the insurgents won.

As strange as it may seem today this brutal and inhuman penalty was a lenient and philanthropic form of expression for that era, because it was enforced in order to limit the death penalty, without the emperors or insurgents, as the case might be, losing sight of their main goal which was the removal to a safer distance of the dangerous foe from the throne or the crushing of every ambition to covet it. The penalty of blinding and also the 'custom of amputation', as Professor Karayiannopoulos [1987] notes, 'at least as far as Byzantium is concerned, was enforced not as an instance of barbarous ethics and inhumanity, but with a deeper constitutional rationale. As is well known, according to Byzantine imperial reasoning, only the best man might aspire to be emperor. But what constitutes the best? Herein lies the importance of bodily integrity and soundness of limb. The mutilation of a limb meant that this individual was deprived of a vital qualification for ascending the throne, for theoretically an amputee was considered handicapped and under no circumstances could he look to the imperial throne and authority.' This view is documented by Zonaras who referring to the blinding of Leo Phocas and also that of his son Nicephorus, writes: 'Brutally they put their eyes out with the result that they lost both their happiness and their lust for kingship or imperial authority' (Zonaras 3, 538, 12–14). Indeed according to this Byzantine conception the penalty of blinding proved tremendously effective. Throughout the history of the Byzantine empire there was only one instance of a blind emperor ascending the throne, that of Isaac II Angelus, who ascended the throne with his son Alexius IV (1203–1204), after Alexius III was overthrown by the Crusaders. The same rationale lay behind the custom in Persia, its place of origin, where Kavādh, on ascending the throne, blinded the former king in order to proscribe any possibility of his returning to power (Theophanes 97, 15–19; Lampsidis 1949).

Later his son, Hosroes enucleated one of Zamou's eyes 'who was next in line for the throne by reasons of seniority' (Procopius 193, 19–20). The same historian confirms that the blinding of one eye or the destruction of the eyelids and the resulting ugliness comprised, according to Persian custom, an insurmountable obstacle for anyone aspiring to the throne (Procopius I, 50, 18–21 and De Bello Gotthico 505, 19–22, 506, 1–4).

It is not the object of this study to ennumerate in minute detail the hundreds of instances of blinding which are mentioned in Byzantine historical texts and which in any case are presented at length in more specialized studies (Lampsidis 1949). Our study is limited to analyzing certain instances, which are of interest from the medical standpoint.

For a start it must be remarked that the penalty of blinding was enforced in one or both eyes by an executioner and his assistant without any particular care being taken. This is made clear by the chroniclers and by illustrations which are, however, later than the relevant manuscripts [Grabar & Manoussacas 1979].

There were three types of blinding practised by the executioners:

A. *The destruction or removal of the eyes by mechanical means*. The destruction or preferably the removal of the eyes was usually achieved by an iron dagger. When an executioner had no dagger available, he would use any sharp tool. Cedrenus, for example, mentions the use of iron tent pegs, Psellus a kitchen knife, Pachymeres fence pegs and finally Anna Comnena mentions a candelabrum (Cedrenus 2, 703, 6; Psellus 1, XLIX, p. 81, 3; Pachymeres 1, 425, 10–12; Anna Comnena, 1, 14, 29–30).

B. *The destruction of the eyes by fire (heat)*. (a) Burning or charring of the eyes, using a heated iron or other tool or more rarely 'burning coals' (Lampsidis 1949). The method is named 'blinding by fire' (πήρωση) and eyes blinded in this manner called 'fire-blinded' (πεπηρωμένα). The method was originally practised by the Persians, who it seems, passed it on to Byzantium. The blinding of Zami by Hosroes, mentioned earlier, followed this method (Phocopius 1, 193, 18–19). (b) Less frequently the eyes were destroyed by using boiling liquid such as oil or vinegar. This method, like the former, has Persian origins as Procopius asserts (De Bello Persico 1, 33, 4–10).

C. *The destruction of the eyes by combined methods, more rarely with a sharp heated instrument*. This method was also known to the Persians, as attested to by Theophylactus: 'iron nails heated in a charcoal fire were poked into the iris of the eye' (170, 22–23, 171, 1–2).

Several examples of ways of destroying the eyes and their results are taken from the writings of Byzantine historians and chroniclers to be examined and approached regarding the medical problems which follow.

A. *The mechanical destruction of the organ of vision*

The enucleation of the eyes with an iron instrument was practised to a great extent, even as a preventative measure against suspected revolt by Constantine VIII (1025–1028). Psellus remarks, in relation to this, 'regarding those suspected of plotting to ascend the throne he instantly blinded their eyes with an iron instrument' (Psellus 1, XXV, p. 25, 8–11). This method which is generally known as severing (εκκοπή) by the Byzantine chroniclers and amounted to the surest method of complete and total blinding was particularly preferred by Michael Paleologus who imposed it on a large number of his victims (Pachymeres 1, 24, 6–11, 2, 154, 18–19, 1, 484, 5–20, 1, 487, 3–8, 493, 7–15, 2, 229; Gregoras 1, 201, 17–19). Basil I (867–886), when he captured the Thracian general Symbatios and the general of the Theme of Opsikios Piganis, who led the revolt against him, also blinded them by this method (Theophanes Continuatus 241, 1–16, 263, 13–18; see also Grammaticus 247, 22–23, 248, 14; Symeon Magister 680, 8–23, 681, 1–3; Georgius Monachus 834, 10–16; Cedrenus 2, 201, 4–6, 205, 16–21; Skylitzes 134, 81).

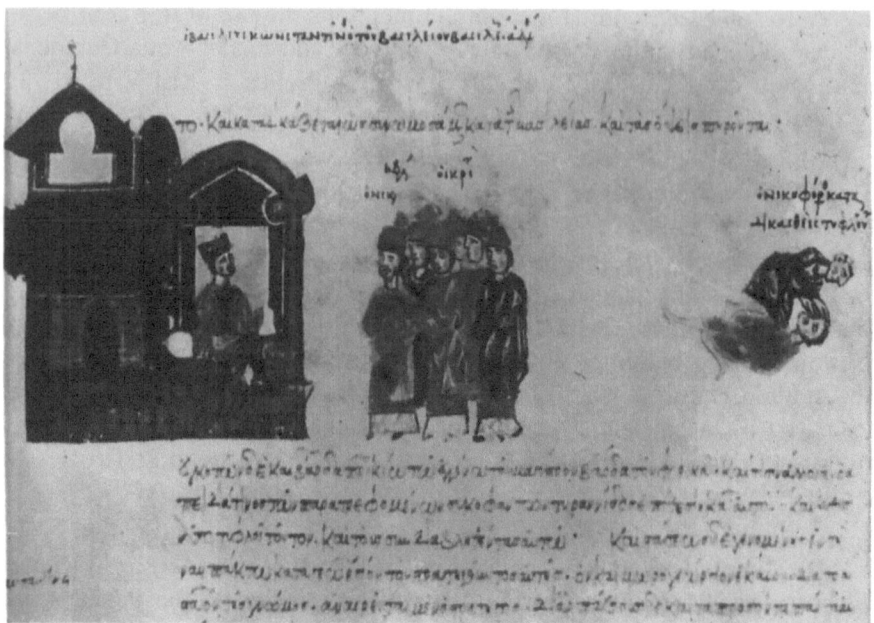

Fig. 1. The blinding of Nicephorus during the reign of Constantine VIII (1025–1028). Chronicle of John Skylitzes (Madrid Library, Grabar and Manoussacas 1979).

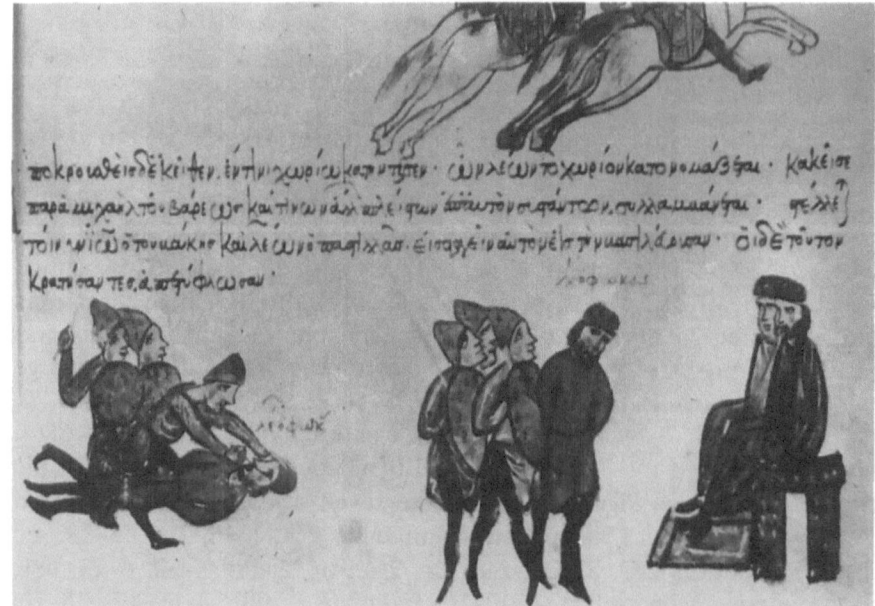

Fig. 2. The blinding of Leo Phocas after his rising against the young king Constantine VII Romanos Lecapinos (920–944). Chronicle of John Skylitzes (Grabar and Manoussacas 1979).

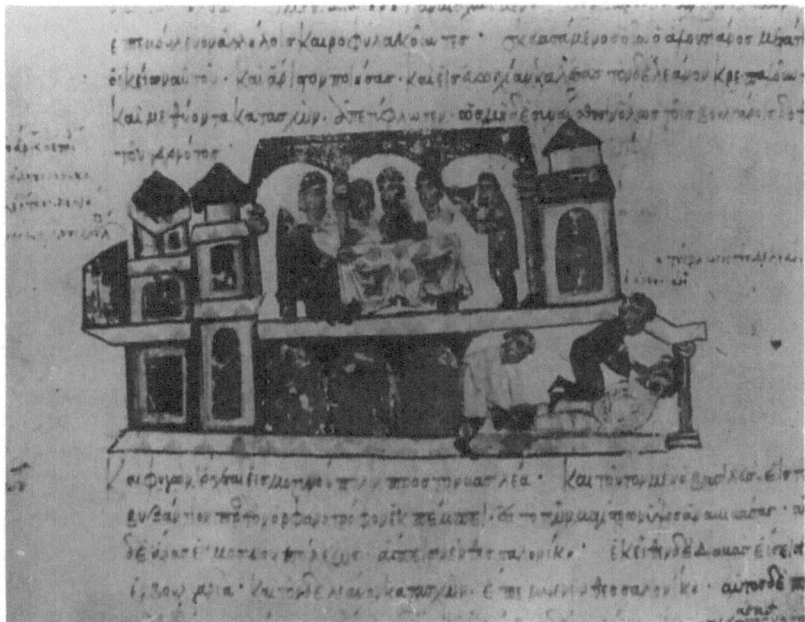

Fig. 3. The blinding of Deleanos under Michael IV (1034–1041). Chronicle of Skylitzes (Grabar and Manoussacas 1979).

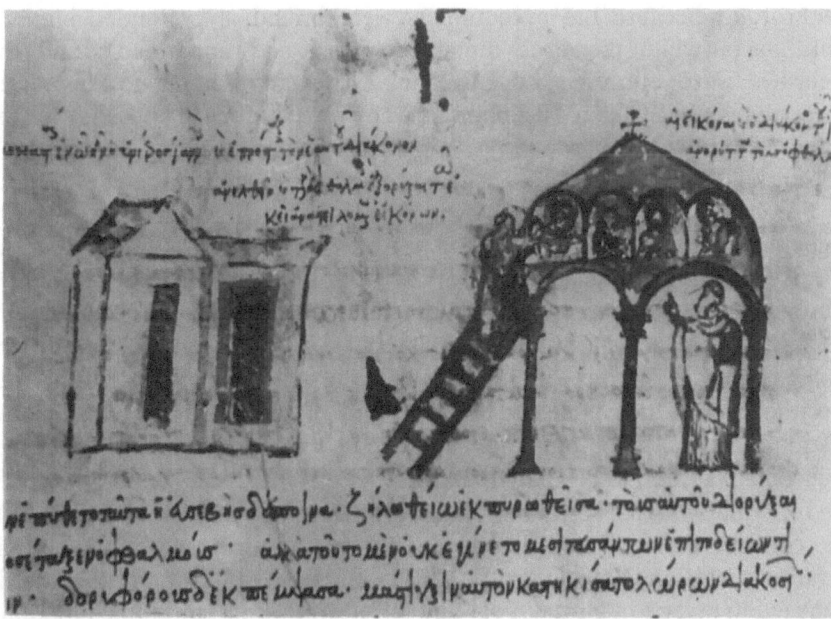

Fig. 4. The destruction of eyes in the icons (!), an expression of the iconoclast climate (Grabar and Manoussacas 1979).

B. *The destruction of the visual organ by fire* (*heat*) (Πήρωση)

(a) *Using a red-hot burning tool.* The emperor Isaac II Angelus (1185–1195) came to the Byzantine throne after the dethronement and the tragic death of Andronicus Comnenus and practised the penalty of blinding by fire to a great extent, his sons Andronicus I, John and Manuel being his first victims (Choniata 466, 11–19, 472, 7, 553, 16–18, 554, 8–11, 556, 20–21, 561, 1, 572, 14, 560, 13–14). But divine justice was satisfied, as it were, in his case as he himself was finally punished with the same penalty in the Monastery of Vira when he was overthrown by his brother Alexius III (1195–1203), so that he was thereafter led by the hand, having undergone blinding by fire (Choniata 727).

The Byzantine chroniclers describe dozens of instances of the fire penalty (Cedrenus 201, 4–6, 213, 5–8, 296, 5–7, 531, 3–7, 550, 23–24; Acropolita 6, 5–6; Pachymeres 375, 9–11; Choniata 408, 1–2; Genesius 8, 18–20, 10, 7–9; Attaliota 17, 11–14). From the wealth of these references we will examine those which occupied the chroniclers to a greater extent for from these descriptions, many useful conclusions may be arrived at.

A characteristic example is that of the blinding of Leo Curopalates and his son Nicephorus, who were arrested under John Tzimisces (969–976) as initiators of the revolt against him. The emperor for reasons of philanthropy, despite the judgement of the death penalty ruled by the court of justice, granted their lives, ordering their exile to Methymna in Lesbos and the penalty of blinding instead of death. Either due to a new order by the emperor, or because the executioners were bribed, a pretended blinding took place (while the eyes remained whole and unharmed), and the eyelashes were burned. Leo Diaconus writes in relation to this: 'Leo Curopalates and his son Nicephorus, who were sentenced to death by the court, were however pardoned by a philanthropic decision of the king who did not kill them. After he sent them to Lesbos he blinded the eyes of both by fire' and 'Leo Curopalates, who was guarded together with his son, Nicephorus, in Methymna, Lesbos, as I have mentioned, after bribing the guards with gold proceeded to revolt, with his eyes intact. For the executioner formerly charged with blinding him, burned only his eyelashes and left his pupils intact and this he did *either* at the orders of the king, for it is implied, and the proof is that later, despite the evil events that followed, the executioner was not punished for any one of them, *or* because the executioner himself pitied him and was moved by his (Leo's) great misfortune' (Diaconus 114, 12–16, 145, 10–20, see also 147, 20–22, Zonaras 3, 525, 12–16, 538, 3–14, Cedrenus 2, 389, 8–18, 404, 12–14, Skylitzes 292, 21). The condemned men, according to the information provided by the chroniclers, did not appreciate the mercy of the emperor and bribing their guards managed to escape in a small boat and to return to Constantinople intending to foment a new rebellion. After this relapse the emperor arrested them anew and this time blinded them completely.

Constantine IX Monomachus (1042–1055) also had many blinded by this method. When he ascended the throne, he called to Mytilene, for reasons of revenge, the man who was responsible for his sufferings, the eunuch John the Orphanotrophus and blinded him by fire: 'the eunuch John, who became the Orphanotrophus, the brother of King Michael Paphlagonus, when the Monomachus reigned as emperor, had John's eyes destroyed by fire after he was transported to Mytilene. And some believe that this was at the order of Queen Theodora without the knowledge of the emperor. And some others say that since the order for this was given by the same emperor because he hated the Orphanotrophus for having formerly exiled him (i.e. the present emperor) without good reason. The Orphanotrophus lived a few days after the blinding and then died (Zonaras 624, 14–19, 625, 1–2). The death of the victim after a few days is characteristic in this case and apparently due as will be more fully analyzed below, to hardship and the possible infection of his wounds. The penalty of blinding by fire was also used to punish Michael Anemas, the instigator of the conspiracy against the life of the emperor, Alexius I (1081–1118).

This penalty was finally revoked: 'A new conspiracy was quickly formed against the emperor, headed by Anemas, Michael, aided by many who were officers in the army. But before they managed to proceed to specific action their movements became known and they were arrested so that their beards were stripped off, not with a razor, but with a plaster mask of pitch (δρώπαξ). Anemas, himself, was left with head and chin untouched but also sentenced to blinding. While the discoverers of the conspiracy were enjoying the fruits of this triumph, a royal decree arrived excluding Anemas from the penalty and revoking the decision to remove his eyes. After confiscating their property, they were sentenced to exile, each one to a different place' (Zonaras 745, 9–20).

More familiar and characteristic are the incidences of the blinding of Bulgarian captives by Basil II the Bulgar-Slayer (976–1025). As is well known, the captives were blinded pitilessly by the thousands and for every hundred blinded in both eyes, one man was blinded in one eye in order to lead them to the king of the Bulgars, Samuel who on seeing the tragic sight, fainted and soon died. The description of Glycas, here following, is characteristic: 'The king after blinding the captive Bulgars, who were said to be approximately fifteen thousand and after ordering every hundred of them blinded by heat in both eyes to be led by a one-eyed man, sent them to Samuel. He was unable to bear the pathetic sight, grew dizzy, fainted and fell to the earth (Glycas 578, 2–7; see also Cedrenus 2, 458, 14–16, 462, 24).

Michael VIII Palaeologus (1259–1282) used this penalty as an exception in order to blind the young John Lascaris whose throne he usurped. It appears that either because, during his reign the penalty had fallen into disuse, or further, for reasons of philanthropy he chose blinding by a red hot drum (ηχείο) which was held close to the eyes of the victim. This last blinding in Byzantium, which is doubted by many, is mentioned by Phrantzis as follows: 'Some who sympathized with the other faction spoke of the penalty Michael the king, his great-grandfather put upon John Lascaris by blinding him and taking his kingdom' (Phrantzis 41, 16–18). From the information provided by historians it is clear that blinding by fire was usually done by putting the heated iron tool in the eye in such a way that the eye was totally destroyed. This appears to be what Choniata infers when describing the blinding of Seth Sclerus, he refers to the characteristic sizzling sound (σίδηρος σίζων) of the red-hot iron which comes into contact with water or a wet surface ('the hissing of the iron' 192, 16). In any case the characteristic preparation of the iron tool which is described by Psellus (1, p. 114, 8) is that of heating it till it was red-hot. The same method was referred to by Procopius as well (De Bello Gotthico 2, 505, 17–22 and De Bello Persico 1, 33, 8–10) and by Simocatta (170, 23 and 171, 1–4).

(b) *Blinding by boiling liquid.* Less frequent was the pouring of boiling liquid (usually oil or vinegar) into the orbits. In this manner Andronicus Palaeologus and his son John were blinded. Ducas refers to this blinding when he writes: 'For Andronicus had only one eye open while John, his son, could see with both eyes by squinting, though he was also cross-eyed,' (Ducas 46, 4–6, see also Ducas 44, 17–19 and Chalcocondylas 60, 18–22, 61, 13–14, 46, 1–2).

This manner of blinding and not only this one, was particularly preferred by Andronicus I Comnenus (1183–1185 A.D.), who Nicetas Choniata characterizes as a hater of sunlight, (μισοφαή) and this is plainly what he infers when he writes: 'Oh how many eyes you blinded with burning liquid' (383, 21).

(c) *Other means of blinding.* Pretended and false blinding were a special type of the penalty of blinding of no particular medical interest. Using the first, the eyes were covered by firm material which was named a 'blinding cloth' (τυφλοπάννιν), and stamped with special seals whose removal was forbidden. Plainly this pretended blinding was imposed for a certain period of time (Lampsidis 1949). From Anna Comnena also we read of the false blinding of Urselius during which the executioners pretended to execute and the victim pretended to undergo the penalty of blinding without its actually having been done: 'And he lay on the earth and the executioner brought the iron tool to his eye and he roared and sighed exactly like a lion. All this an apparent deprivation of the eyes (the pretended blinding) and the supposedly blinded man had been informed to shout and cry and the executioner had been instructed to look at him wildly and to use mad gestures in such a manner so as to convey a more authentic performance of the pretended blinding. So that he was 'blinded' without being blinded and the executioner ranted, raved and everywhere announced the blinding of Urselius' (Anna Comnena 1, 14, 29–30, 15, 1–8).

Conclusions. In summation we conclude that the penalty of blinding in Byzantium was enforced by various means and in order of frequency,

(a) by destroying or enucleating the eyes with a sharp instrument,

(b) by fire held close to the eyes and finally,

(c) by pouring a boiling liquid in the eye orbits.

The first way was more certain to achieve total blinding because it brought on a complete destruction of one or both eyes, and in the case of both eyes being blinded, the complete destruction of vision (visual acuity zero). That the penalty of severing is heavier as compared with the penalty of blinding by fire is attested to by the words of Georgius Cedrenus, who, regarding the blinding of Leo Phocas and his son, Nicephorus notes: 'the king, wanting to use them more mercifully, condemned both to permanent exile and blinding by fire, by mistake it is said, as the king ordered the executioners not to destroy their eyes at all, but to give the impression of having blinded them, while in fact they kept their sight. The king further ordered them to conceal that this order was his own so that it seemed that the executioners were merciful philanthropists who granted the condemned men their vision' (Cedrenus 2, 389, 11–19).

It is characteristic of the executioners to enforce this penalty with violence which many times led not only to the destruction of the eyes but also to the protective parts of the eye, e.g. the eyelids and the adjacent tissues. Ducas' description is typical. He writes: 'They so gouged and scraped his eyes that no trace of the eyelids or skin remained' (186, 7–8). Attaliota, also referring to the blinding of Diogenes Romanos by some clumsy Jewish executioner writes: 'And they permitted some unpractised Jew to proceed in blinding the eyes. And they tied him from four sides and tied his chest and belly and many fell upon him to hold him . . . and they brought the Jew who put out his eyes most painfully with an iron tool, while the victim below roared and bellowed like a bull and no one pitied him. And when this was repeated (the action with the iron tool) his punishment was ended . . . and his eyes were finally destroyed and their liquid spilled. When he rose his eye orbits filled with blood, truly a pitiful and deplorable sight, bringing unbearable sorrow to those who saw him, half dead, finished also from the disease he had. Then he was sent seated on a humble animal until he arrived at the Sea of Marmara. He dragged himself, exactly like a rotten corpse with his eyes put out and his head and face, from which grubs or worms appeared and fell, were swollen. After he lived several days in pain and exuding a bad odour, he finally died and was buried on the island of Proti, on the mountain peak . . . leaving the memory behind him that his troubles surpassed even Job's' (Attaliota 178, 10–23, 179, 4–11, 15–17).

It must be regarded as certain that after blinding, no precautions were taken to avoid infection, at least on the part of the executioners or more generally by the torturers. The binding of the eyes after blinding with special bandages, which is mentioned by Anna Comnena, was not to prevent infection but for the sake of appearances. That is, in order to cover the deformity caused by the usual careless blinding practises. This is plainly implied by the remarks Comnena makes in the *Alexiad*: 'symbolic bandages appeared on eyes which had apparently been blinded' and 'wearing the symbolic bandages of blindness' (Anna Comnena 1, 15, 20–21 and 1, 16, 1–2).

Under these circumstances of blinding, the resulting infections were often a common cause of the death of the victim. A characteristic example are the instances of the eunuch John the Orphanotrophus, already mentioned and of Diogenes Romanos whose head and facial tissues, according to the descriptions of the chroniclers became infected with an inflammation resulting in worms as well as in an evil odour, a situation which quickly brought on his death on the island of Proti. Zonaras' description, despite his tragic subject, is particularly elegant: 'The king's order that he be blinded was sent there and his eyes were immediately put out in the presence of the bishops. His eyes were removed in a crude manner and without the necessary care so that an oedema, a swelling of the head resulted and the wounds bore worms and the air about him was rank with the odour of infection. In this ugly and ill condition he was transported to the island Proti . . . and after living there briefly, died and was buried there' (3, 706, 1–19). But the description of Glycas does not lack elegance either and is equally dramatic (612, 17–21, 613, 1–2).

Other chroniclers refer to the tragic death of Diogenes Romanos (Ioannes Curopalates 704, 18–23, 705, 1–2; Attaliota 175, 15–23, 179, 4–11, 15–17; Tsolakis 1958; Skylitzes Continuatus 154, 14; see also Karayiannopoulos 1977). Apart from the infection of the tissues surrounding the eyes it was very likely that the endocranial infection spread through the tunics of the carelessly injured optic nerve forming an endocranial abscess, and further creating the more general septicaemia born of the extensive infection of the tissues. These infections and their results explain the notable number of victims who are mentioned by the Byzantine historians as dying after blinding. Mentioned among them is Constantine VI who had the unbelievable and tragic ill fortune to be blinded by the order of his own mother, Irene. This dramatic event which created such a grievous impression on public opinion that it was connected with a chance eclipse of the sun is described by Theophanes: 'And towards the ninth hour they blinded him in a painful and incurable manner in order that he die, in accordance with the decision of his mother and her advisors. The sun was dark for seventeen days and shed none of its rays so that the ships wandered and all men said the sun hid its rays because of the blinding of the king; and thus Irene, his mother, reigned' (732, 5–11; see also Cedrenus 27, 13–18, Pétridés 1900–1901, Brooks 1900, Misiou 1980). Though Constantine finally survived, the penalty of blinding led to the deaths of John Orphanotrophus, John Comnenus the son of Andronicus I, Theologos Corakas, Lambros and others (Cedrenus 550, 23–24; Lampsidis 1949).

With the two other methods of blinding, that is by fire and by pouring 'heated liquid', the executioners were able to achieve a controlled blinding, i.e., the incomplete blinding of the victim. This was easily achieved either by regulating the temperature of the heated iron or the boiling liquid, or by holding the heated tool closer to or further from the eyes or finally by regulating the amount of liquid poured on the eyes. The case of Leo Curopalates and Nicephorus is mentioned as typical. In this case the executioners held the red-hot iron tool at such a distance so as to burn only the eyelashes. The blinding of John Lascaris is also interesting. Pachymeres describes this event in detail: 'And the child whose age was just beyond the age of babyhood is denied its vision and in this only the executioners showed mercy, in that when they executed the abominable deed they did not destroy the eyes with an iron tool but with a drum which was heated and which they brought before the eyes of the youth. This in order to char his eyes which withered in the heat and also that his visual faculty might dim gradually (ηρέμα) (Pachymeres 1, 191, 20, 192, 1–6). According to this detailed description by Pachymeres it is clear that a heated iron was not used, for this would cause total blindness. But a heated drum, was held close to the eyes and this dried them out or withered them apparently creating a small leucoma of the cornea and a small drop in visual acuity, that is partial blindness. It is characteristic that in using the word 'gradually' in this case, which might be interpreted to mean, 'quietly', 'lightly', 'slowly', the partial loss of vision is plainly implied in point of fact (Stamatakos 1972). Conversely in the case of pouring liquid, highly heated, or even in the case where the heated tool came into direct contact with the eyes so as to be termed 'sizzling' by historians, then it is certain that total blindness of the victims followed. A characteristic example is the penalty of blinding by fire in the case of Isaac Angelus which resulted in total blindness because, as Nicetas Choniata asserts, when he was restored to the throne with his son Alexius, 'he assumed the royal throne led by the hand because he had suffered blinding by fire' (Choniata 727; Lampsidis 1949; Karayiannopoulos 1977).*

With the adjustments mentioned above the executioners permitted the victims to retain a working vision, in most cases (since for reasons of humanity they wished to inflict only partial blinding), and at other times a visual acuity, characterized in ophthalmology as useful (up to 6/20), something which could not be achieved in the case of severing or by the destruction of the eyes. These conclusions are supported by the fact that in cases where those ordering the penalty, hoped for total blinding, the execution of the order was assured in an oath by the executioners, as in the case of the blinding of Romanos IV Diogenes, which has been mentioned already (Attaliota, 178, 17–20).

---

* We must also take note of a well-aimed psychological remark of Nicetas Choniata, which we often come across in our patients today, that is that Isaac Angelus, believing in oracular prophecies, hoped to regain his vision (Choniata 737, 14).

144

The wealth of information provided by Byzantine historians and chroniclers about the inhuman penalty of blinding, so much favoured and widespread among the Byzantines, beyond its legal interest, also provides illuminating facts for the subject to be approached from a medical standpoint.

References

1. Anna Comnena. Annae Comnenae Porphyrogenitae: Alexias. Ed. Augusti Reifferscheidii, Vol. I. Lipsiae: Bibliotheca Scriptorum Graecorum et Romanorum, Teubneriana, 1884.
2. Brooks WE. (1990). On the date of the death of Constantine, the son of Irene. Byz. Zeitschrift 1990; 9: 654–657.
3. Corpus Scriptorum Historiae Byzantinae. Editio emendatior et copiosior, consilio B.G. Niebuhrii C.F. (50 vols. Bonnae. E. Weberi 1828–97). The references quoted refer to the volumes with the titles: Constantinus Manasses-Ioel-Georgius Acropolita, Michael Attaliota, Theophylactus Simocatta-Genesius, Georgius Monachus, Michael Glycas, Leo Grammaticus-Eustathius, Ducas, Ioannis Zonaras, Theophanes, Georgius Cedrenus Vols. 1 and 2, Ioannis Curopalatae, Leo Diaconus, Nicephorus Gregoras, Georgius Pachymeres Vols. 1 and 2, Procopius 1: De Bello Persico, Procopius 2: De Bello Gotthico, Symeon Magister- Pseudosymeon, Theophanes Continuatus, Georgius Phrantzis, Laonicus Chalcocondylas, Nicetas Choniata.
4. Grabar A, Manoussacas IM. (1979). L'Illustration du manuscrit de Skylitzès de la Bibliothèque Nationale de Madrid. Venice: Institut Hellénique d'Etudes Byzantines et Post-Byzantines de Venise.
5. Karayiannopoulos I. (1987). History of the Byzantine State, Vol. 2. Thessaloniki: Vanias Editions.
6. Lampsidis O. (1949). The Penalty of Blinding by the Byzantines. Doctoral Thesis. Athens.
7. Misiou D. (1980). Irene and Theophanes' Term 'Paradoxically'. Contribution to the 'Constitutional' Position of the Byzantine Augusta. Byzantina 10: 171–177.
8. Pètridés S. (1900–1901). Quel jour Constantin, fils d'Irène, eut-il les yeux crevés. Echos d'Orient 4: 72–75.
9. Psellos Michel. (1926). Chronographie ou Histoire d'un Siècle de Byzance (976–1077), Vol. 1 Paris: Ed. Emile Renauld (Société d'Edition 'Les Belles Lettres').
10. Skylitzae I. (1973). Synopsis Historiarum. Corpus Fontium Historiae Byantinae, Vol. 5. Berolini.
11. Stamatakos I. (1972). Dictionary of the Ancient Greek Language. Athens: Phoenix Editions.
12. Tsolakis E. (1958). A Continuation of the Chronicle of John Skylitzes. Thessaloniki.
13. Vasiliev A. (1932). Histoire de l'Empire Byzantin, Vol. 2. Paris.

Address for correspondence: Dr John Lascaratos, 9 Oreinis Taxiarchias St., Zographou, Athens 15772, Greece.

Documenta Ophthalmologica **81**: 145–152, 1992.

Miraculous ophthalmological therapies in Byzantium

JOHN LASCARATOS
Athens, Greece

Key words: History of ophthalmology, miraculous cures, Byzantium

Abstract. A series of cures for ophthalmological diseases practised by saints are described, particularly the Saints Cosmas and Damian and the Saints Cyrus and John, the famous 'Anargyroi'. In the xenones of the Byzantine churches and in the hospitals connected to these, therapeutic regimes, cures and surgical interventions took place at night during incubation, following the example of the ancient Asclepieia. This conclusion stands in spite of the fact that the authors describing the lives of the saints were often clergy who frequently cloak the true therapeutical cures by presenting them in a supernatural manner in order to stress the divine intervention of the saints. From the operations mentioned, it is clear that cataract surgery was among the operations most frequently practised.

Studying the lives of the saints is interesting in regard to the history of medicine during Byzantine times [3, 18, 28]. After Christianity took over, the work and activities of the healing gods of the national pantheon, such as Asclepius, Amphiaraos, the Dioskouroi and others were replaced by various saints, such as Theodore, Artemios, Febronia, Minas, Demetrius, Therapon, Pantelaeimon, Nicholas, Thecla and others, especially the pairs of physician-saints known as *anargyroi*.[1] According to Runciman's acute observation [28], 'the many monks and hermits who were famous for their therapeutic abilities were not alone, for the Christian churches had inherited the beneficial offices which formerly belonged to the idolatrous temples'. From the study of the lives of the saints we may conclude that the hospitals (xenones) were usually found beside the churches and particularly those churches dedicated to the Anargyroi, i.e. to the Saints Cosmas and Damian, and Cyrus and John. The two most important religious centres of the East dedicated to the Anargyroi, were in the Patriarchal churches of Antioch and Alexandria. They were largely the scene of surgical and pharmaceutical therapies for various illnesses.

The most important of the four churches of Constantinople dedicated to Cosmas and Damian, was the famous Monastery of Kosmidion, built in ca. 440 AD by Paulinos, the favourite magister of Theodosius II, famous from the apple anecdote. The monastery was renovated by the emperor Justinian, in gratitude for his cure by the holy doctors. The monastery provided lodging for worshippers and care of the sick. It also was used for surgery and

---

[1] They were called Anargyroi, because they did not accept payment for their cures. In Greek, the word *anargyros* refers to a person extending a service free of charge.

housed a school for doctors. The historian Procopius writes that the church of Cosmas and Damian was founded at the inmost point of the Kerateios (Golden Horn), where once Justinian was cured of a dire disease after the doctors had given him up. The same historian also notes that when the doctors were unable to cure patients, the patients would cross the Kerateios in boats and make for the Monastery of Kosmidion where they would find refuge in the temple of the Saints Cosmas and Damian [27]. In the famous temple of Kosmidion, the Bishop Laurentius of Lychnis was cured of a physical disability. He returned to his home where he lived to be over eighty years of age, according to Marcellinus [20]. According to the chronicler Paschale, the monastery was set on fire by the Arabs in 626 AD [32].

Therapy in the temples acquired a miraculous character and took place at night during incubation. While the patients slept in the temple or in the xenones, the saints appeared in a dream and revealed the manner of therapy. The Saints could also realize a cure by miracle or by a bloodless, i.e. pretended surgical intervention, or finally by actual surgery. It is clear that the priests and the rest of the medical staff of the xenones used the same therapies which had come down from the priests of the ancient Asclepieia. This phenomenon of incubation amounts therefore to an ancient tradition of the Asclepieia. It must be noted that it has been retained until even our times in various churches in Greece on the festival day honouring the saint of the church. On such a day incubation of the sick could be observed awaiting holy grace to be cured by a miracle [21, 25, 31, 32]. From the information provided by various historical sources and especially from manuscripts surviving from the xenones [8–12] it is certain that ophthalmological diseases received conservative treatment in the xenones of Byzantium, but we may assume that in the xenones surgery was performed too, as was described by Paul of Aegina [13] and Leo the iatrosophist [17]. The latter recommends couching of the cataract, not in its early stages but when it has advanced. Further information on the treatment of cataract is confusing, though it is clear that most therapies tend to be conservative and not surgical. Another surgical therapy of patients suffering from hernia is known to us from the Miracula Sancti Artemii [25], which proves the surgical pre-occupations of the doctors in the xenones. It seems very likely that the doctors must have been occupied with cataract operations as well. Furthermore, there is specific evidence which documents these suppositions.

In a relevant cure (E10)[2] of the Saints Cosmas and Damian, the case of the writer and orator, Stephanos of Tarsos is mentioned [32].* It is clear that in this case the operation for cataract took place with a *kentitirion*.

---

[2] The letter C before the number of the cure refers to those mentioned in the Constantinople collection. The letter E refers to the manuscript of Edfu, while the letter A refers to the cures of Saints Cyrus and John [5, 29, 32].

* He was blind for five years and he was an inmate of the Kosmidion monastery awaiting treatment. After his eyes had been pierced and pricked by an iron tool by the doctors of the monastery he regained his sight.

In cure numbered E27, two patients are described who suffered from epichysis (cataracts). It is said that the saints obliged one of them to borrow and buy poultry for his food, while residing at the temple, for he was poor. Despite this he was not cured and he protested because he was forced to borrow money. The second patient, also suffering from cataract, was wealthy. The saints on the strength of a vision ordered him to pay 120 coins to the poor patient in return for his cure. This was a sizeable sum for those times as the coins were gold. The rich patient did indeed pay the money to the poor patient who was arrested by the guard when he stepped outside the monastery to relieve himself. The guard slapped him thinking he was escaping with the money. From this slap his sight was restored as well as that of the rich patient who grew frightened when he heard the poor man's cries. This cure can be interpreted as the abrupt or sudden dislocation of the cataract lens from the slap to the poor man, but does not explain the cure of the rich man unless it was not a case of cataract but of some other eye disease. It is sufficient however to understand that this description serves to praise the therapeutic successes of the saints. We come across similar instances in the hand down descriptions of the cures of the ancient Asclepieias. It was clear that the physician-saints saw to it that the rich worshippers practised philanthropy in favour of the needy.

A cure which refers to the well-known popular theme of a trial of purity is contained in cure C25. Among the worshippers there was a patient suffering from ophthalmia. The saints revealed to him that he would be cured if he bathed his eyes with the milk of a sensible and prudent woman. Indeed the milk of such a woman who had come to the church with her husband was used. Her husband, 'driven by the devil' was jealous and in this manner the purity of his wife was proven. This cure recalls the ancient remedy of Egyptian medicine, the urine of a virgin, but also the milk which was used until recent years in the Greek countryside as a popular cure for eye ailments.

As a cure, purely to stress the miraculous ability of the saints, as well as a threat or warning, we encounter cure C43. In this case the shepherd of the monastery, who was sent away by the monks, tried to set fire to the stable. The saints prevented him and he went blind. He regained his sight only after he expressed his repentance. This miracle reminds us of similar miracles of the ancient Asclepieias.

Other interesting cures, though usually without a scientific explanation, are the cures of Saints Cyrus and John which are described by the monk Sophronius [30]. The main category of their cures consists of miracles, though surgery is never mentioned even for the sake of appearances.

The bedevilled blind man of cure A65 was cured of blindness by driving out the devil which caused the blindness. Demons are often cited as a cause for blindness and accounted for one third of the cases cured by the saints.

We know from the book by the Bishop Georgios of Alexandria entitled *Concerning St. John Chrysostom*, that in the Monastery of St. John a certain

Eucleos, who lost his right eye through the power of a demon, retired to the monastery to become a monk. While he was cutting his hair in preparation for his ordination and was praying to the saint, his eye was miraculously cured [26].

It is of interest and this also proves the high frequency of eye diseases in Egypt at that time, that Sophronius' 17 cases, i.e. approximately 20% of the total, refer to ophthalmological diseases.[3] Sophronius also mentions an inscription of gratitude donated to the church by a Roman worshipper, Cure A69. He was cured by the Saints without either the cause of his eight year blindness being mentioned or the method of therapy. Plainly this therapy had significance as propaganda.

Two blind men of Cure A46 were cured after carrying out the orders of the Saints to wash out their eyes in the pool of Siloam of Jerusalem, known to us from the Bible. A man suffering from leukoma in cure A2 was ordered by the Saints to wash out his eyes in the church spring. When he had done so he saw the leukomas fall out into his handkerchief. In the cures of Saints Cyrus and John the therapy for cataract is mentioned only as a conservative treatment. In cure 51A Georgios the Presbyter, possibly suffering from cataract, was cured when he applied cerate (κηρωτή) and cheese to his eyes as advised by the saints. We must clarify that the saints prescribed cerate as a panacea, a sort of thick ointment which was made of wax from the candles lit in the church. Cerate was often used for the therapy of ophthalmia and blindness in the form of a plaster.

Even the author, the monk Sophronius, who suffered from cataract himself, was cured, as he later writes, after many visions in which he saw Saints Cyrus and John, Saint Theodore and the Apostle Thomas. He used the oil of the saints' lamps to anoint his eyes (Cure A70). The blind woman of Cure A24 received a curious instruction from the saints in a dream. She was to roast crocodile meat and grind it to a powder. She was to apply this to her eyes and in this manner she regained her sight. In order to cure leukomas in Cure A47 the sufferer received the following command. He was to go to the bath of the church and bath his eyes with white-wash diluted in water. This cure is curious because the saints cured someone with a caustic substance which could have blinded him. In four cures the malady was enforced as a punishment, as in the patients of cures A37 and A38, who were blinded with leukomas because they were heretics. Or in the cases of the patients of cures A28 and A31 because the first was an astrologer and the second a blasphemer. The blasphemer, A31, was blinded for cursing after Holy Communion and was cured by the Saints after he repented. After a three-day period of waiting in the church he saw the burning coals in the

---

[3] Ophthalmological diseases were widespread at this date and not only in Egypt. John of Ephesus notes that in the streets of Amida there were many blind and disabled unfortunates to be found at the side of the road, ignored by all men [18].

censer during the liturgy. In the cure A28, two blind men were cured. One, the astrologer Nemesion was blinded because he believed, like all of his kind that the heavenly bodies are gods. It is plain that he was cured by the saints and this is mentioned indirectly because he subsequently carried out the marble work and icon painting of the saints' tombs. The poor blind man in the same cure was cured when Nemesion, acting on the orders of the Saints touched his eyes.

In cure A37, a sufferer of leukomas of the cornea, saw a vision of the saints seated before their tomb. They ordered him to drink a glass of milk and gave him some bread. He explained this as an order by the saints that he adhere to Orthodoxy, which he did and was cured. He subsequently repented of this decision and returned to his heretical misconceptions and the saints blinded him with a slap. When he repented anew and returned to the church, he regained his sight when the deacon read the phrase, 'he had been blind and received his sight' (St. John 9: 18) from the Bible.

It is clear that these cures have a proselytizing and terrifying character. The same point lies behind Cure A38, where another heretic suffering from the same disease saw the saints offering him the Host which fell from his hands. He also interpreted this correctly to mean that he must take Communion and alter his views with the result that he was cured. When he too returned to heresy, he was blinded anew. And he repented again when he saw Christ and the church in a dream. Finally he was cured by washing his eyes with the juice of a weed, *cichorium*.

Another patient A9, sceptical of the cures of the saints, was cured by them of ophthalmia from which he suffered when he saw a vision of the church, the saints and a crowd of worshippers.

In the church of Saint Theodoros in the Egyptian city of Diolcus, St. Nicholas Sionites met the blind man Antonios. Antonios complained that he had spent all his money on doctors without regaining his sight. St. Nicholas assured him that as long as he believed in the saints he would be cured. And he was cured the very next day for Saint Theodoros took oil from a vigil lamp of his own church and anointed his eyes making the sign of the cross [18].

According to the *Ecclesiastical History*, Evagrius [1] mentions the miraculous cure of a wounded eye. Specifically he refers to the wife of Arkesilaos, a patrician ruler of a city in Palestine. She had hit her eye with the shuttle of her loom in such a way that the pupil of the eye had fallen out as the eye had been cut completely across. In those days, John the Ascetic, a contemporary of Zosimas, lived by the wall of Houziba which was located at the northern point of the avenue joining Jerusalem to Jericho. When he was sent for and saw the wound, John the Houzibite asked the doctors who had gathered to bring a piece of sponge with which he replaced the contents of the eye into their socket as much as possible. He left the sponge on the wound and subsequently tied it with a wide linen bandage. Arkesilaos was not present but was with ascetic Zosimas, who seeing him cry and weep, went to the adjacent room to communicate with God. Then he came to Arkesilaos saying, 'the grace of God was granted to the Houzibite. Your wife has been cured and is well in both eyes'. Although the second part of this story by Evagrius stresses the presence of miraculous therapy, we must not overlook that in effect a surgical operation took place. The contents of the eye socket were replaced and the wounded eye restored [1, 18].

Other characteristic examples are the miraculous cures by Saint Thecla which are mentioned during her life [4]. Among the multitude of miracles noted, many cases of ophthalmological cures are described. Specifically it is noted that when a pandemic of ophthalmia afflicted Isaurian Seleucia during the summer 'and a very severe rheuma from the head bore towards the eyes and therapy by the doctors was impossible (the doctors being at a loss and perplexed in such cases), the martyr opened her surgery in the church where the afflicted would assemble to be cured'.

Another well known case is that of a highly distinguished patrician from Cyprus who was blinded. According to the prevalent rumour he used a drug prescribed by the Saint and returned to his home cured, with his vision restored. Another case which is mentioned is that of a poor labourer, Pausikakos, who suffered from a disease of the eyes and was blinded by the neglect and clumsiness of the doctors. With the help of Saint Thecla he regained his sight. Another case concerns the disease of a baby which 'due to much weeping, displayed a serious problem in one of its eyes.' Established medicine could not cure him so his nurse brought him from Olva in Isauria to the neighbouring city to Saint Thecla's church (Martyrion). As a result, the eye recovered, the child was cured and regained his sight. His father Pardanios and his grandfather Anatolios who was the priest of the Olva church marvelled at his cure [4].

From these descriptions we must conclude that the xenones of the churches fostered a situation where miracles took place side by side with actual medicine as is the case with the cures of the Asclepieia. Generally speaking we can maintain that from a medical standpoint the major interest of the cures lies in the pharmaceutical therapy prescribed, or the dietary regime or the surgery, even if fictitious. Of interest too are the cures where the supernatural element plays a part for they help us to study the mentality and superstitions of the Byzantines. Given also that medicine in that era could offer limited help, many natural cures which are found among the cures of the saints and are attributed to miraculous intervention, are certainly due to the healing processes of nature herself [31].

We cannot accurately assess in figures or percentages to what degree these therapies are due to fictitious or actual operations, or to the faith of the patients as to whether their visions were genuine or a product of their imagination. Or finally whether a deliberate presentation of anecdotes by the chroniclers of the cures was meant to exaggerate the miraculous powers of the saints.

It would be excessive of course to believe in certain operations such as the removal and cleansing of the intestines of a patient suffering from bulimia or the transplant of a leg of a dead man to replace the amputated limb of a patient of Saint Cosmas and Damian.

In any case it follows that actual operations were performed by the doctors of the monastery accompanied by the blessings of the saints. It is also clear that the doctors of the monastery, who represented a personification of Saints Cosmas and Damian, performed cataract operations [32]. Further it must be stressed that the majority of the cures by Saints Cosmas and Damian had a scientific basis in contrast to the Egyptian cures of Cyrus and John, where the medical basis appears weak and is often ridiculed by the monk Sophronius, as most illnesses are attributed to demonic factors and medicine is powerless to expel the demons or dissolve the magic. Most of the medical prescriptions mentioned, such as cerate or oil from church lamps or crocodile meat or camel stool have very little to do with true pharmaceutical action. Among the true medicines only aloe is mentioned [32]. Surgical interventions are not mentioned by the Egyptian Anargyroi, although bloodless treatments such as massage are. These differences stress the different cultural level between the two pairs of Saints and indicate the superiority of the Anargyroi of Constantinople who had both a Greek education and a good medical knowledge [32].

In conclusion we can discern the true medical treatments from the large number of cures for ophthalmological diseases mentioned in the lives of the various saints. We can separate the true medical care provided from the superstitions and the exaggerated stress laid on the saints' therapies as well as from the incomplete references to the medical or surgical therapies the patients underwent during incubation while staying at the xenones of the church. From studying the writings on miracles we conclude that these xenones were the scene of pharmaceutical and surgical interventions provided by the staff and aimed to cure ophthalmological diseases.

References

1. Bidez J, Parmentier L. (1898). *The Ecclesiastical History of Evagrius*. London: Methuen and Co.
2. Codellas PS. (1942). The Pantocrator, the Imperial Byzantine Medical Center of XIIth Century A.D. in Constantinople. Bull. Hist. Med. 12: 392–410.
3. Constantellos DJ. (1986). Byzantine Philanthropy and Social Welfare. Athens: Ed. Phos.
4. Dagron G. (1978). Vie et Miracles de Sainte Thècle. Text Grec. Tr. F. Commentaire. Brussels: Société de Bollantistes.
5. Deubner L. (1907). Kosmas und Damian. Leipzig-Berlin.
6. Gautier P. (1974). Le typicon du Christ Sauveur Pantocrator, Revue des Etudes Byzantines 32: 1–145.
7. Koukoules Ph. (1957). Byzantine Life and Civilization. Athens: Collection de l'Institut Français d'Athènes: VI.
8. Kousis A. (1928). Contribution à l'étude de la Médecine des Zénons pendant le 15ᵉ siècle basée, sur deux manuscrits inédits. Byzantinisch-neugriechische Jahrbücher 6: 77–90.

152

9. Kousis A. (1944). Manuscripts. The Apotherapeutic of Theophilos According to the Laurentian Codex. plut. 75, 19. Proceedings of the Academy of Athens 19: 35–45.
10. Kousis A. (1944). Manuscripts. Les oeuvres médicales de Nicéphore Blémmydès selon les manuscrits existants. Proceedings of the Academy of Athens 19: 56–75.
11. Kousis A. (1944). Medical Manuscripts. The Medical Work of Romanos According to the Vatican Greek codex 280. Proceedings of the Academy of Athens 19: 162–170.
12. Kousis A. (1944). Medical Manuscripts. The Written Tradition of the Works of Leo the Iatrosophist. Proceedings of the Academy of Athens 19: 170–171.
13. Lascaratos J, Marketos S. (1982). Cataract Surgery in Ancient Peoples. Ophthalmological Annals 19: 121–147.
14. Lascaratos J, Matsagas A, Marketos S. (1987). Therapy In Byzantine Hospitals. New Information for the Cure of Ophthalmological Maladies. Bulletin of the Hellenic Ophthalmological Society 56: 162–166.
15. Lascaratos J, Tsirou M. (1990). Ophthalmological Ideas of the Byzantine Author Meletius. Documenta Ophthalmologica 74: 31–35.
16. Lascaratos J, Tsirou M, Fronimopoulos J. (1990). Ophthalmology According to Aetius Amidenus. Documenta Ophthalmologica 74: 37–48.
17. Leon, Philosopher and Physician. Synopsis of Medicine. Anecdota Medica Graeca. Lugduni Bavatorum: Pub. FZ Ermerins, 1840.
18. Magoulias HJ. (1964). The Lives of the Saints as Sources of Data for the History of Byzantine Medicine in the Sixth and Seventh Centuries. Byzantinische Zeitschrift 57: 127–150.
19. Malalas, Ioannes. (1831). Chronographia. 304–306. Bonn: Corpus Scriptorum Historiae Byzantinae.
20. Marcellinus Comes. Monumenta Germaniae Historica (MGH), AAXI, 99. Berolini: 1877–1898.
21. Marketos S, Fronimopoulos JN, Lascaratos J. (1989). The treatment of eye diseases in the Asclepieia. Documenta Ophthalmologica 71: 155–165.
22. Miller TS. (1983). Byzantine Hospitals. Dumbarton Oaks Symposium (Byzantine Medicine): 53–63.
23. Miller TS. (1985). The Birth of the Hospital in the Byzantine Empire. Baltimore/London: The Johns Hopkins University Press.
24. Orlandos A. (1941). The Reconstruction of the Xenon of the Monastery of the Pantocrator in Constantinople. Epetiris of the Society of Byzantine Studies 17: 198–207.
25. Papadopoulos-Kérameus A. (1909). The Miracles of the Glorious Miracle Worker and Saint, the Grand Martyr, Artemios (Miracula S. Artemii). St. Petersburg: Varia Graeca Sacra, 1–79.
26. Photius (1960). Bibliothèque II. Paris: Société d'Edition 'Les Belles Lettres'. Tr. R Hendry.
27. Procopius (1838). De Aedificiis. Ed. Weber. Bonn: Corpus Scriptorum Historiae Byzantinae II, Vol. III, 193.
28. Runciman S. (1969). Byzantine Civilization. Trans. D. Detzortzi. Athens: Galaxias-Ermeias.
29. Rupprecht E. (1935). Cosmae et Damiani, Vita et Miracula. Berlin: Neue Deutsche Forschungen.
30. Sophronius. (1860). Encomion Cyrus and Ioannis. Ed. J. Migne. Paris: Patrologia Greca 87: 3389–3418.
31. Toole H. (1963). Asclepius, Part I: Asclepius in History and Legend. Surgery 53(3): 387–400.
32. Toole H. (1975–1976). The Miracles of the Physician-Saints Cosmas and Damian (Anargyroi). Epetiris of the Society of Byzantine Studies 42: 253–297.

Address for correspondence: Dr John Lascaratos, 9 Oreinis Taxiarchias St., Zographou, Athens 15772, Greece.

Documenta Ophthalmologica **81**: 153–161, 1992.
© 1992 *Kluwer Academic Publishers.*

Interview

The development of ophthalmology
in the former German Democratic Republic after 1945

RUDOLF SACHSENWEGER
Leipzig, Germany

Key words: History of ophthalmology, German Democratic Republic

Introduction. In an interview with the editor of this issue, H.E. Henkes, held in the autumn of 1991, Prof. Sachsenweger describes the developments in the field of ophthalmology which took place in East Germany after World War II. He is particularly able to do this because, to my knowledge, no other chairman of a department who worked in the German Democratic Republic (GDR) during several decades without affiliation to the ruling communist party (SED), and as a politically independent citizen, suffered from so much opposition and obstruction. This report necessarily reflects a personal view; no doubt younger colleagues will be able to paint the picture in greater detail, on the basis of historical documents that hopefully in the future will become available. (H.E.H.)

H.E.H.: *What was the situation with regard to eye care in the former German Democratic Republic?*

R.S.: After the war, patient care in the Soviet-occupied territories of Germany returned to normal surprisingly quickly, because many older ophthalmologists continued in their former private practices and the optical industry soon recovered to a large extent from war damage and partial dismantlement.

A fair number of colleagues moved to West Germany very soon after the war, not only because of the far better career opportunities and stabler conditions of life, but also because of the uncertainty and obstruction with respect to the higher education of their children. In the Federal Republic of Germany they made good the losses in our specialty caused by the war.

Up to 1961, the year in which the Wall was built, East German ophthalmologists who completed their training settled with few exceptions in West Germany.

After 1961 it became increasingly difficult and unrewarding to pursue private practice in the GDR. Many older colleagues sought a position in a state-owned health centre, mainly in order to secure a pension. The low payments made by the public health services compelled ophthalmologists with a private practice to treat large numbers of patients. After 1961 no one could open a private practice, and only exceptionally were the children of physicians allowed to continue their parents' practice.

Ophthalmologists working in health centres found that their initiative and efficiency were not rewarded. Their career advancement was hampered by party regulations and a vastly overblown bureaucracy.

The health centres contributed to the loss of prestige of medical doctors. The union FDGB was the physicians' official representative, but it operated primarily in the interests of the communist party; professional associations were strictly forbidden.

The chief medical officer of each province (*Bezirksarzt*) allotted a certain number of graduate students to the various universities and provincial clinics each year. He acted as the superior officer of all physicians in a province, i.e., of the medical practitioners of approximately one million citizens. He organized, supervised and exerted political control. The directors of clinics, sometimes even of university clinics, depended on his whim and fancy. He was – after the Minister of Health – the highest state official and always a proven, absolutely reliable, member of the Party.

If the director of a clinic was able to create an atmosphere which inspired confidence, many assistants wanted to stay on after their final examinations. In most cases the application was granted. If however the assistants, for whatever reason, wanted to leave the clinic directly after the examinations, the lack of staff could become very depressing.

The health centre system was established and developed primarily for economic reasons; it apparently also served the purpose of discouraging private practice. Obviously it was easier to introduce socialism and political indoctrination into the health system within such a centre than outside it. The politically conformist doctors in such a system were automatically at an advantage with respect to promotion, honours and titles.

Departments of strabismology were instituted much later in East than in West Germany because of lack of the equipment which had to be imported. For a long time there were far too few qualified orthoptists. They were vastly underpaid, so that many left their jobs after their training period. The founding of schools of orthoptics in Greifswald and Leipzig was delayed until 1961 by bureaucratic obstacles. The original concept had to be curtailed, in particular in respect of the amount and quality of the equipment.

The so-called 'Government Hospital' in Berlin deserves special mention. It was established for the benefit of high Party and State officials, for their parents and their children. Since these persons, who were documented in a secret catalogue, were usually elderly people, treatment of the grandchildren of these privileged civilians on the spot was not possible.

The Government Hospital in Berlin, like the special health centres for the police and the army, was far better equipped than the general health centres with regard to imported drugs and instruments, even if the latter were not fully utilized. The staff of the Berlin Government Hospital was four times the size of that of the general health centres and twice the size of that of the hospitals for the police and the army. The medical activities of the physicians in the Government Hospital were absolutely secret, as was everything in connection with this institution.

Physicians working in the Government Hospital received unusually high salaries: they were specially selected on the basis of their political reliability and absence of relatives or friends in West Germany or any contact or correspondence with West German citizens. Party members in high positions and so-called 'anti-fascists' also received special treatment.

Up to 1965 the population was adequately supplied with optical glasses. After 1965 the typical symptoms of a centralised command economy appeared. In order to obtain certain types of glasses, a wait of 6 to 12 months became necessary. This fact was particularly depressing because, before the war, nearly the entire German optical industry had been concentrated in the East, in Jena and Rathenow. Very few satisfactory intra-ocular lenses were available before 1990, so that surgeons had to persuade cataract patients to try to obtain their intra-ocular lenses abroad.

In the 1980's the number of ophthalmologists was nearly sufficient. Waiting periods were due largely to the inherent inefficiency and insufficient organisation of the out-patient departments. Moreover, bureaucracy, time wasted in getting the necessary materials, and especially the employment of medical specialists for non-medical tasks, were responsible for a substantial loss of efficiency and satisfaction.

Doctors were delegated to military exercises and to participate in summer camps and party and union courses of instruction. Much time and energy were absorbed by the so-called political-ideological, marxistic-leninistic courses (monthly indoctrination courses in the clinics, regular courses in political instruction, party schools, etc.).

In spite of all this, the population by and large was adequately cared for, thanks to the dedication and hard work of the ophthalmologists and the proximity of the medical standards set by West Germany.

H.E.H.: *What was the situation regarding the training of ophthalmologists?*

R.S.: The quality of the ophthalmological training programme differed greatly from clinic to clinic. After 1961, the head of the clinic had little or no influence on the selection of graduate medical students. The distribution of the graduates over the universities was made by the ministry and by the chief medical officer of the province. Neither the choice of the clinic director nor of the graduates was considered. Frequently, the head of the clinic was only informed just prior to the start of the training period on the number of graduates he might expect and who they were. Those students who had direct or indirect Party connections (members of the SED or the so-called Block Parties) had a far better chance of receiving the training of their choice than their colleagues. Graduates also had better chances if their fathers had political connections. At the beginning of his residency, each doctor was informed which health centre he would later be assigned too.

During the ophthalmological training period, each graduate student had to follow mandatory courses in military and social medicine, organized by the chief medical officer of the province or by the Berlin Academy for Continuing Medical Training. At that academy, as well as at the University and the hospitals of the Medical Schools, one or two 'refresher courses' were given annually, free of charge. Neither in quality, nor in quantity could these arrangements compare with the abundant choice of study courses and congresses arranged for ophthalmologists in West Germany. None the less these courses not only met the needs of their East German counterparts, but produced a level of knowledge which, according to nearly all ophthalmologists who emigrated to West Germany, came up to the qualifications needed to comply with West German standards.

From the late 1950's, a State Board examination followed the residency. In the early years, the final examinations were held in the university eye clinics, not supervised by State officials. Later on, they were centralised in the Berlin institute, and included questions on military and social medicine and on Marxism-Leninism. Training courses also existed for nurses, headnurses, orthoptists, medical-technical assistants and other para-medical personnel.

The standard German textbooks (a.o. by Axenfeld-Pau, and Velhagen) were available in sufficient quantities. The textbook by Axenfeld-Pau, although it was relatively expensive, was imported at long intervals, but other West German and foreign publications became available only sporadically and in insufficient numbers.

In theory, the supply of textbooks to students was sufficient, but as new editions, even of popular student's textbooks, were published only after great delay owing to paper shortage and bureaucratic failure, it often happened that students bought all copies of a new edition immediately after publication and stored them away at home.

Modern educational methods (audio-visual equipment, video films, etc.) were not available; similarly, a working knowledge of English was hard to attain. In spite of mandatory eight-year courses in Russian at school, students were far from mastering the Russian language. Some directors of eye clinics arranged courses in English for their assistants.

Medical study reforms led to successive shortening of the time allotted to lectures and laboratory work in ophthalmology for the sake of education in Marxism-Leninism, military medicine and hygiene. In the end, it became practically impossible to cover the entire field of our specialty during the training period. Doctors passing the State Board examination in ophthalmology were not required to demonstrate proficiency in ophthalmic surgery, a serious disability for those wishing to practise in West Germany. They had to find a colleague prepared to teach them the operations needed to obtain a licence as ophthalmic surgeon in West Germany.

H.E.H.: *What developments took place in the field of ophthalmological research?*

R.S.: Before 1961, the standard of ophthalmological research in East Germany was more or less comparable to that in West Germany. After 1961, it declined precipitously and finally fell behind by a decade. To a large extent, this was the result of the mediocrity of the newly-installed chairmen, whose nomination was influenced by Party dominance and Party politics. The composition and quality of the faculty was certainly not the result of natural, ideology-free selection, a problem which will carry on into the future.

After the retirement of three heads of departments and the death of a fourth, only two of the nine chairs of ophthalmology were occupied by professors free of Party connections. The authorities were prejudiced against independent candidates: one of them, for instance, was passed over twice in favour of a SED-member. Before 1961 an independent candidate was occasionally appointed, because qualified candidates were at that time extremely scarce as hundreds of ophthalmologists had either left the country or chosen not to pursue an academic career but to settle in the provinces. Before 1958 a West German professor was appointed to the chair in one of the GDR-universities, but when he was called to a chair in West Germany, his successor was a Party-member. The appointment to a chair in ophthalmology was more often than not the result of negative selection, never a natural, ideology-free choice. Nevertheless, in every specialty some non-Party members were appointed, in order to support the pretence that equality of opportunity existed.

Even now, after the overthrow of the regime, former Party members still form the majority on many boards: some enjoy a certain esteem in foreign countries because of a reputation earned thanks to former profitable arrangements connected with Party-membership. As many of the old structures in reality still exist, there is a real danger that foreign colleagues will not be aware of the connection of these members with the former SED.

Permission to travel to scientific meetings abroad was only granted to reliable party members (*Reise-Kader*). As a result, certain SED-members became known in the West, although neither their scientific output nor their integrity justified this. The participation in meetings in Western countries was used as a means of demonstrating their political integrity; insufficient information meant that many Western colleagues accepted the suggested picture.

Another reason for the scientific decline was the lack of modern scientific and clinical equipment and the forced isolation of young East German scientists. Financial resources for the importation of instruments from the West were totally insufficient. The Ministry of Health and the Party grotesquely demanded that scientists should orientate their research on the standards set by the Soviet Union and its satellite countries. The Party slogan was: 'Learning from the Soviet Union means learning to win'. Opportunities to travel to East-block countries and to the USSR were rarely made use of.

Readers of Western scientific journals were gradually forced to cancel their subscriptions. In 1962, all directors of eye clinics were ordered to make sure that all existing East German memberships of the (West) German Ophthalmological Society (DOG) were cancelled, although no membership fees had ever been levied. Each month the chief medical officer of the province had to be informed about the cancellations.

Annual DOG-Congress reports were no longer distributed, not even to retired members of the Society. Even the mailing of films of a purely scientific nature was forbidden. After 1980, two professors, almost always the same two, were allowed to attend the annual meetings of the DOG. Only very rarely were East German colleagues, who had been invited in person by the DOG, granted permission to attend.

The infiltration in committees of international societies by party members was also an objective. The election of a representative of the GDR to the Board of the European Ophthalmological Society (EOS) may serve as an example. After the death of the representative, a successor had to be elected. The authorities proposed three politically reliable party members, although all three were unknown to the Board of the EOS. For this reason I was elected. Consequently there was great difficulty in getting permission for me to participate in the annual Board meetings of the Society, even in the years (1980 to 1984) of my presidency! In this period, the Board convened in Paris in connection with the centenary of the French Ophthalmological Society. Permission to leave the country however, was not granted on the pretext that the French Consulate did not have enough application forms for permission to enter France. But a personal visit to the French Consulate revealed no lack of forms whatever. This initiative, however, resulted after some weeks in a reproval by the president of the university on the grounds that no GDR-civilian was allowed to enter a foreign embassy without the consent of his superior.

The election of a new representative of the German Democratic Republic to the Board of the EOS met with similar obstructions: three reliable Party-members were placed on the list; nevertheless, the Board chose a non-Party member who was mentioned by the authorities only in the fourth place.

The award of the Von Graefe Prize by the (West) German Ophthalmological Society to me in 1967 resulted in a two-hour interrogation in which members of the State Security Service (the notorious *Stasi*) tried to press me to renounce the prize, which the East German authorities considered to be a form of bribery or reward. Only the fact that I was at that time the president of the Ophthalmological Society of the German Democratic Republic prevented them from pressing their point further.

For non-Party members, the bureaucratic red tape involved in planning travel abroad was formidable: one had to fill in a multi-page form eight times. The most important questions concerned the fulfilment of political objectives. The applicant had to detail the manner in which the political aims of the GDR could be furthered and the export of goods facilitated. He had to explain in what way the experiences gained abroad would serve the State. The form had to be signed by the *Sektionsdirektor*, the director of foreign affairs and the Rector of the University. On returning from abroad, a report in eight copies had to be produced. A brief, preliminary report had to be delivered three days after the traveller's return; the final, detailed report, in which the scientific and political benefits had to be stressed, was due a few weeks later. The traveller was also compelled to report any unusual interest taken in his person; any contacts with persons who had left the GDR at an earlier date: any private invitations or gifts; any attempts to persuade the traveller to leave the GDR or to disobey the laws of the GDR; any political discrimination; any attempts at bribery and any cooperative activities with partners from socialist countries. For someone who was not a Party member, it was not too difficult to use meaningless terms and noncommittal phrases. It was clear that one copy of these 'reports' reached the Secret Service (*Stasi*).

Directly after the war, a subscription to a West-German ophthalmological journal was allowed, but soon after 1961 the authorities pressed for an East German periodical. It took many years, however, before publication of the *Folia Ophthamologica* finally started in 1976. From then on, authors from the GDR were strictly instructed to publish their results only in *Folia*. Continuation of a subscription to the West German *Klinische Monatsblätter für Augenheilkunde* was made quite difficult. The quality of the contributions and the lay-out of the *Folia* could in no way compete with the West German journals. The small number of foreign subscriptions was a perpetual worry to the East German authorities.

Permission to publish abroad was granted very rarely and only to Party members. In the last few years restrictions were lifted slightly. In all respects the authorities wanted to isolate the GDR from West Germany.

The time available to young scientists for research was very limited, as the daily routine of patient care absorbed all their energy. Equally disturbing was the impossibility of obtaining current literature. All young colleagues realized that their professional advancement depended less on the quality of their scientific output than on their proven Party loyalty. In consequence, the scientific mediocrity of a great many young ophthalmologists was understandable. Nevertheless, some non-Party members managed to reach a much higher standard, although for them much greater dedication was necessary. Clearly, this was also true for other disciplines besides ophthalmology.

It is surprising that in spite of all these political restrictions, remarkable achievements were realized, at the price of great effort and enormous perseverance. This holds true especially for the basic medical care of the population; this was far better than in the other socialist countries. Noteworthy is the publication of several ophthalmological handbooks and monographs. They did not represent actual advances in ophthalmology but nonetheless served our field. The most eminent examples are the two editions of the 12-volume handbook *Der Augenarzt* [The Ophthalmologist] by K. Velhagen in which the chapters by Badtke and Tost ('Development and Malformations of the Eye') and by Münchow ('History of Ophthalmology') are outstanding. In addition to this handbook, extensive monographs were written on Internal medicine and the eye, Paralysis of the external eye muscles, Neuro-ophthalmology, etc. Furthermore, excellent clinical research took place on the radiation therapy of ocular tumors and on cryomedicine. The printing and publishing tradition in Saxony, existing from time immemorial, was certainly partly responsible for this activity.

H.E.H.: *How much influence did the Party (SED) have on the ophthalmologists?*

R.S.: The influence of the SED on all medical institutions was enormous and grew stronger and more comprehensive over the years. In every larger clinic an official Party-secretary was active, in addition to largely unrecognized unofficial Stasi-collaborators, who kept watch on the clinic's director, the administration and every single physician; naturally, their aim was to secure the position of the SED. The influence of the Party-secretary reached out to all the activities within the clinic; very few events escaped his attention. He had the power to grant or withhold permission for pay increases, honours and awards, the purchase of equipment, etc. He was assisted by Party-members, in some cases even by the director of the clinic (*Comrade Director*, or *Comrade Professor*), who had to report on the implementation of Party-principles in the clinic. An independent professor was usually left in peace, but had to live with the feeling that next to him a mighty undercover organisation existed which was continuously watching him. In every clinic there was also a Party-bound union secretary who was politically rather inconspicuous.

The Society of East German Ophthalmologists had a General-Secretary who exerted both control and initiative: most often this office was held by a university professor active in Party-politics, and that over several decades.

When certain important questions were being debated at the board meetings, a representative of the general secretariat of all the medical societies in Berlin would be present. When in the 1950's and 1960's several non-aligned professors belonged to the Board, Party-members would meet separately before all meetings to define their course of action in conformity with Party-dictates. Otherwise, for whatever reason, some Party-bound professors were quite tolerant in private conversations, as long as political issues were avoided.

New appointments to university chairs reflected almost exclusively Party interests: Party-members had an absolute advantage. The same applied to the appointment of directors of provincial hospitals and of assistant professors.

In the Ministries of Health and Education, many people in leading positions were vastly underqualified for their jobs. It is understandable that, for this very reason, they pursued uncompromisingly and with great energy the interests of the Party.

There is no doubt whatsoever that, after the reunification of the two Germanies, the former power structures of the SED continue to exist, still undiminished in the universities. It is to be feared that the same persons continue to exert power as interest groups to this day, not only within the university, but in all other realms of society as well.

H.E.H.: *In your opinion, what is the future outlook for East-German ophthalmology?*

R.S.: Great effort will be required to redress the harm wrought by the SED upon ophthalmology in East Germany, particularly by its provincialism. Above all, those persons should be rehabilitated who withstood corruption by refusing membership of the SED in spite of great disadvantages to their careers.

Ophthalmology in East Germany will undoubtedly adjust to the level of ophthalmology in the West within a few years, and thus yield yet another proof of the superiority of a free political order to dogma, dictatorship and incompetence. To attain this goal, all the negative relics of the dominance of the SED-party will have to be removed: the ill-advised appointments, dictated by Party or political interests, will have to be reconsidered.

Address for correspondence: Prof.em. Dr.sc.med. R. Sachsenweger, Heinzelmannweg 12, O-7030 Leipzig, Germany

Stereoscopic Acuity in Ocular Pursuit of Moving Objects

DYNAMIC STEREOSCOPY AND MOVEMENT PARALLAX: RELEVANCE TO ROAD SAFETY AND OCCUPATIONAL MEDICINE

by

Matthias and Ulrich Sachsenweger

Despite the fact that dynamic stereoacuity is of considerable relevance to everyday life, the subject has so far never been systematically studied and is still a blank space on the maps of ophthalmology and physiology. This is equally true for dynamic stereoscopy in binocular vision as well as for perception on the basis of movement parallax, a phenomenon of differentiated contour displacement within a given field of vision which is also available to the monocular individual under conditions of head or body or object movement within the visual space.

This treatise provides a wealth of useful information on spatial three-dimensional perception of moving targets. It is a valuable, informative study on dynamic visual acuity and offers clues for testing and evaluation to readers who are particularly interested in the two modes of dynamic stereoscopic vision. Furthermore, it will prove helpful in providing encouragement for further investigations on dynamic performance of the visual organ.

From the Contents:
(1) Introduction / (2) Elements of dynamic stereoscopic vision: Monocular dynamic visual acuity - Stereoscopic vision - Dynamic parallactoscopy - Experimental factors of stereoscopic vision - Dynamic vision / (3) Equipment and methods for testing dynamic stereoacuity / (4) Normal values of dynamic stereoacuity / (5) Variations of test objects and testing methods/ (6) Dynamic stereoacuity in response to changes in perception conditions/ (7) Effect of psychosensorial factors: Fatique - Effect of psychosedatives - Effect of hypnotics - Short-time and long-time exercises - Asthenopia / (8) Comparison between dynamic and kinetoparallactic stereoacuities / (9) Conclusions / Bibliography / Subject Index

1991, 134 pages - Paperback ISBN 0-7923-1486-7
Reprinted from *Documenta Ophthalmologica*, Volume 78, Nos 1-2 (1991)

KLUWER ACADEMIC PUBLISHERS - DORDRECHT / BOSTON / LONDON

A. BRINI / P. DHERMY / J. SAHEL

Oncology of the Eye and Adnexa
ATLAS OF CLINICAL PATHOLOGY

The authors have put together, side by side, clinical and histopathological aspects of the various neoformations likely to be encountered in eye pathology, including those most recently discovered as well as those most frequently met with. The aim of the authors is to provide their colleagues with a reference MANUAL, conceived so as to permit rapid access to essential concepts in current eye oncology. Rapid and easy consultation of this atlas has been made possible through the use of a comprehensive set of 64 plates, with 375 full-colour figures, with concise accompanying texts in English, French and German, and a detailed index.

From the Contents:
A. Tumours of the eylids and the conjuctiva / Tumeurs palpébro-conjonctivales / Geschwülste der Augenlider und der Bindehaut
B. Orbital and orbito-palpebral tumours / Tumeurs de l'orbite et orbito-palpébrales / Orbitale und orbito-palpebrale Geschwülste
C. Tumours of the uvea / Tumeurs de l'uvée / Geschwülste der Uvea
D. Tumours of the retina and the optic disc / Tumeurs de la rétine et de la papille optique / Geschwülste der Netzhaut und der Papille
Technical appendix / Appendice technique / Technischer Anhang
Literature / Littérature / Literatur
Alphabetical index of subjects / Index des sujets / Sachwörterverzeichnis

Not only students beginning with work in ophthalmology, but also experienced ophthalmologists will find this atlas most useful. At the same time, it should be considerable assistance to pathologists and dermatologists and to practitioners frequently finding themselves faced with ophthalmological problems.

XX + 154 pages with 375 colour-photographs   HB ISBN 0-7923-0409-8

A PUBLICATION OF
Kluwer Academic Publishers - Dordrecht / Boston / London

Monographs in Ophthalmology

1. P.C. Maudgal and L. Missotten (eds.): *Superficial Keratitis*. 1981
   ISBN 90-6193-801-5

2. P.F.J. Hoyng: *Pharmacological Denervation and Glaucoma*. A Clinical Trial Report with Guanethidine and Adrenaline in One Eyedrop. 1981
   ISBN 90-6193-802-3

3. N.W.H.M. Dekkers: *The Cornea in Measles*. 1981   ISBN 90-6193-803-1

4. P. Leonard and J. Rommel: *Lens Implantation*. 30 Years of Progress. 1982
   ISBN 90-6193-804-X

5. C.E. van Nouhuys: *Dominant Exudative Vitreoretinopathy and Other Vascular Developmental Disorders of the Peripheral Retina*. 1982 ISBN 90-6193-805-8

6. L. Evens (ed.): *Convergent Strabismus*. 1982   ISBN 90-6193-806-6

7. A. Neetens, A. Lowenthal and J.J. Martin (eds.): *The Visual System in Myelin Disorders*. 1984   ISBN 90-6193-807-4

8. H.J.M. Völker-Dieben: *The Effect of Immunological and Non-Immunological Factors on Corneal Graft Survival*. A Single Centre Study. 1984
   ISBN 90-6193-808-2

9. J.A. Oosterhuis (ed.): *Ophthalmic Tumours*. 1985   ISBN 90-6193-528-8

10. O. van Nieuwenhuizen: *Cerebral Visual Disturbance in Infantile Encephalopathy*. 1987   ISBN 0-89838-860-0

11. E.A.C.M. Sanders, R.J.W. de Keizer and D.S. Zee (eds.): *Eye Movement Disorders*. 1987   ISBN 0-89838-874-0

12. R. Živojnović: *Silicone Oil in Vitreoretinal Surgery*. 1987
    ISBN 0-89838-879-1

13. A. Brini, P. Dhermy and J. Sahel: *Oncology of the Eye and Adnexa*. Atlas of Clinical Pathology / *Oncologie de l'Œil et des Annexes*. Atlas Anatomo-Clinique / *Onkologische Diagnostik in der Ophthalmologie*. Vergleichender Klinisch-Pathologischer Atlas. 1990   ISBN 0-7923-0409-8

14. J.J. De Laey and M. Hanssens: *Vascular Tumors and Malformations of the Ocular Fundus*. 1990   ISBN 0-7923-0750-X

KLUWER ACADEMIC PUBLISHERS – DORDRECHT / BOSTON / LONDON